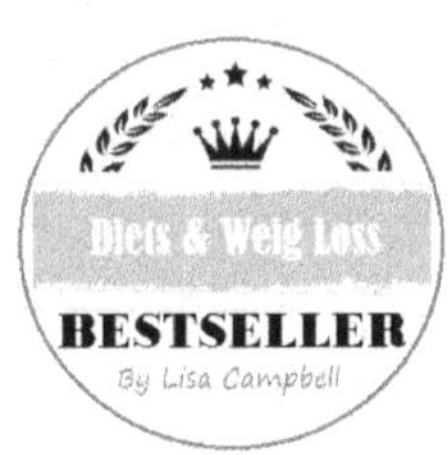

Lose Weight Fast with

Ketogenic Mediterranean Diet Cookbook

The key to lasting health and longevity is yours when you discover the power of the Mediterranean diet combined with a low-carb ketogenic diet!

(2020 Ketogenic Mediterranean Guide)

by Lisa Campbell

© Copyright 2020 by Lisa Campbell

The Ketogenic Mediterranean Diet
Weight Loss Solution

TESTIMONIALS

I have several ATK cookbooks, but this is now our go-to cookbook. It's helped us shift our eating habits away from meat, potatoes and pasta - although all three are included here - to healthier options. I've lost 11 pounds in a month of eating dinners from this cookbook and following their Mediterranean food pyramid.

Annabel - San Diego

This book was recommended by my cardiologist.

I had just had a stress induced heart attack at age 58/female. I don't smoke or drink.

I have lost 30 lbs following these recipes and feel better than ever. Simple to follow and delicious!

Brenda - London

This is an excellent ketogenic mediterranean diet book. From this book you will find lots of healthy and delicious recipes which will help you to lose your weight and lead a healthy life. I really enjoyed this book and found it very educational. After reading this and learn many things. I highly recommended this book! Lovely! Wow! I like it

Divina - Orlando

The ease and use of this book is wonderful for someone who has a family to look after, while looking for nutritious meals for the family that are easy to make. I also found this cookbook easy for people who may have restricted diets and need to alter recipies. I really liked the flavor and ease of this cookbook as well.

Lorainne - Las Vegas

My husband is recovering from trip by-pass surgery and this is the diet recommended by his surgeon and the hospital's dietician. We're enjoying it and modifying it a bit during his recovery to include a little less fat. The book is informational and educational, and it includes a sample 7-day meal plan as well as several recipes. I find it easy to follow, the recipes are clear and easy, and taste really good.

Nicole - New Orleans

This is a wonderful introduction to the Ketogenic Mediterranean Diet. The first few chapters explain the philosophy and details behind the diet and are easy to read. Then the second half of the book are recipes—and the recipes are amazing! I finished the book and couldn't wait to start trying several of the recipes. I can't say enough about how useful this book is—I highly recommend it.

Roxy - Texas

The Mediterranean Diet is an excellent guide for people looking to make the switch to a healthy lifestyle. The Mediterranean diet is not your typical regimen of restricted foods and calorie counting, but rather is a way of eating, exercising, and leading a healthy life. A life that will be less vulnerable to heart disease and certain forms of cancer as made evident by the studies presented in the book from the New England Journal of Medicine. This book serves as a guide that eases you into this lifestyle where food is appreciated, it brings people together, and enriches the bodies of those that consume it. Readers learn how to wean themselves off unhealthy foods and receive recipes with ingredients that can be conveniently purchased at local stores and markets. The recipes are easy to follow making the transition into the Mediterranean Diet, a smooth one.

Roxanne - New York

"This has to be the best diet/cookbook I've ever purchased. The plan is easy to understand and use, the meals consisting of ingredients that are either on hand or easy to find anywhere. There is prep involved, but most of it is easily done within a half an hour, not including cook times. I have a renewed interest in cooking now, feel great, and am losing weight. Most of all, there isn't one dish in two weeks that I haven't enjoyed--if an ingredient (e.g. fennel) isn't what I like, I just pick another meal. This is a life-changing "how to" book!"

TABLE OF CONTENTS

Ketogenic Diet

Mediterranean Diet

Introduction

The current statistics in a world of obesity is frightening, especially when considering the direct correlations to illnesses and diseases. The increases in these numbers are not only affecting Americans but many more countries in the world, according to information from WHO (World Health Organization). Even though these figures are high, people who want to do something about it can, since they have effective regimens like the well-known Ketogenic Mediterranean Diet as a weight loss option.

Current Obesity Trends

Based on the staggering figures from WHO, approximately 2/3rds of all Americans adults can be classed as overweight. All of the high calorie hamburgers, sundaes, French fries, sodas, cheese cakes, ice cream and other popular food items are taking its toll. Even though American maintains the lead, as in many other areas, they are not alone in this problem because many other countries are now following the same patterns. If these current trends are not halted, the prediction for 2030 is nearly half of all Americans may be obese. While this problem is big and massive to the world, the change that occurs can be drilled down to a one-on-one choice. This means, if no one makes a change, it is up to the individual to take the information that they have learned and act on it.

The Ketogenic Mediterranean Diet Is a Lifestyle

Acting on it requires making a change. This change, however, is not finding another fad diet because they can only compound the problems. Instead, it requires making life style changes in the foods that people eat on a daily basis.

This is one of the major benefits to the Mediterranean Life style approach. With a growing body of evidence from the medical world (i.e. Harvard School of Public Health, Dariush Mozaffarian MD. DrPH. and others in the medical community), this diet is known for its numerous health benefits. From helping to prevent diabetes to the protection of cardiovascular diseases, this is a life style change that can help people remain healthy even when they are out socializing with peers and colleagues.

Benefits

The mass acceptance of this life style and its benefits can be confirmed by participants on the Mediterranean Coasts, since they have eaten this way for thousands of years. In this area of the world, it is not a diet plan but it is the way that the vast majority of the population eats. While leading healthy lives with regular exercises, they enjoy a wide range of different foods including yogurt, fish, poultry whole grains, fruits, vegetables, beans, nuts, olives, and olive oil along with some cheeses. The foods that this culture eats are responsible for providing antioxidants, vitamins, minerals, and fibre. All of these elements work in cohesion together to protect the person from all kinds of chronic disease and illness.

The current state of obesity in the world is disturbing because its impact is far reaching. From the increase in obesity to all kinds of illnesses and diseases, this is a problem that is being addressed on many different fronts. However, the ultimate decision to what occurs in the future will depend on each individual, as they choose what to and what not to eat.

So, with that in mind it's important to know that there is a solution to this problem and that is what we will cover in this guide. So without further ado let's dive right in.

CHAPTER 1: WHAT IS KETOGENIC DIET?

The keto diet is a low or zero carbohydrate diet, but it differs from other low-carb diets (such as Paleo) in that it deliberately manipulates the ratios of carbs, fats, and protein to switch fat into the body's primary source of fuel. Our bodies are used to using carbohydrates as fuel. Fats, which is a secondary source of fuel, are rarely tapped on. That means the extra fat is stored and keeps adding on the pounds.

The only ways to reduce fat in a 'normal' diet are to consume less fat and workout a lot in order to increase energy expenditure over daily calories intake, which is why most people fail to lose weight on conventional diet.

On the other hand, the ketogenic diet uses fat for fuel, which means it gets used instead of being stored. So, weight loss becomes easy. In addition to weight loss, the ketogenic diet is known as the "healing" diet. The lack of sugar intake has been proven to help and prevent many diseases such as heart disease, high blood pressure, cancers, epilepsy, and many symptoms of aging.

The manipulation of carbs, fats, and protein is curcial in order to get into ketosis. It's a state when the body, deprived of the usual carbohydrates and sugar, is forced to use fat as its primary fuel. So the ratio of fats and protein are significantly higher than carbs in general.

Of course, consuming less carbs also means lowering the amount of insulin in your body. Less insulin; Less glucose and fat storage. That is why the keto diet has been so successful in helping people with diabetes. It adjusts the sugar level naturally.

The ratio of carbs, fat, and protein can vary. Many people allow themselves up to 50 grams of carbohydrates a day and still lose weight. On a stricter regime, the carb intake can be between 15 and 20 grams daily. The less carbs, the quicker the weight loss, but the diet is very flexible.

On the keto diet, you don't count calories. You count carbohydrates and adjust the intake of carbs vs. fat and protein. A typical keto diet will get 60 percent of its calories from fat, 15 to 25 percent of calories from protein, and 25 percent of calories from carbohydrates. The only limitation on the diet is sugar, which you need to avoid.

The ketogenic diet is not a fad. Many scientific studies have shown the benefits and healing effects of ketosis. Discuss the ketogenic diet with your doctor if you are interested in consuming less sugar, losing weight, or as preventive measures against vulnerable health problems.

CHAPTER 2 - BENEFITS OF KETO DIET

Although ketogenic diet is popularly known as a 'rapid fat loss diet', it is actually more to this than meets the eye. In fact, weight loss and higher levels of energy are only by-products of the keto diet, a kind of bonus. It has been scientifically proven that the keto diet has many additional medical benefits.

Let's begin by stating that a high carbohydrate diet, with its many processed ingredients and sugars, has absolutely no health benefits. These are merely empty calories, and most processed foods ultimately serve only to rob your body of the nutrients it needs to remain healthy. Here is a list of actual benefits for lowering your carbohydrates and eating fats that convert to energy:

Control of Blood Sugar

Keeping blood sugar at a low level is critical to manage and prevent diabetes. The keto diet has been proven to be extremely effective in preventing diabetes.

Many people suffering from diabetes are also overweight. That makes an easy weight-loss regime a natural. But the keto diet does more. Carbohydrates get converted to sugar, which for diabetics can result in a sugar spike. A diet low in carbohydrates prevents these spikes and allows more control over blood sugar levels.

Mental Focus

The keto diet is based on protein, fats, and low carbohydrates. As we've discussed, this forces fat to become the primary source of energy. This is not the normal western diet, which can be quite deficient in nutrients, particularly fatty acids, which are needed for proper brain function.

When people suffer from cognitive diseases, such as Alzheimer's, the brain isn't using enough glucose, thus becomes lacking in energy, and the brain has difficulty functioning at a high level. The keto diet provides an additional energy source for the brain.

A study by the American Diabetes Association found that Type 1 diabetics improved their brain function after consuming coconut-oil.

That same study indicated that people who suffer from Alzheimer's may experience improved memory capacity on a keto diet. Those with Alzheimer's have seen improved memory scores that might correlate with the amount of ketones levels present.

What does this study mean to an average person? With the emphasis on fatty acids, such as omega 3 and omega 6 found in seafood, the keto diet is likely to fuel the brain with the additional nutrients to help achieve a healthier mental state. The brain tissue is made up largely of fatty acids (you've heard fish referred to as "brainfood"), and the increased consumption of those fatty acids will logically lead to improved brain health.

Our body does not produce fatty acids on its own; we can only obtain it through our diet. And the keto diet is rich in fatty acids.

A diet high in carbohydrates can lead to a "foggy" brain, where you have difficulty in focusing. Focusing becomes easier with the increased energy provided by the keto diet. In fact, many people who have no need or desire to lose weight use the keto diet to improve and enhance brain functions.

Increased Energy

It's not unusual, and has become almost normal, to feel tired and drained at the end of the day as a result of a poor, carbohydrate-laden diet. Fat is a more efficient source of energy, leaving you feeling more vitalized than you would on a "sugar" rush.

Acne

While most of the benefits of a keto diet are well-documented, one benefit catches some people by surprise: better skin and less acne. Acne is fairly common. Ninety percent of teens suffer from it, and many adults do, as well.

While it was always thought that acne was at least exacerbated by poor diet, controlled research is still being conducted. However, many people on the keto diet have reported clearer skin. There may be a logical reason. A 1972 study found that high levels of insulin can cause the eruption of acne. Since a keto diet keeps insulin at a low and healthy level, it may very well affect skin health.

In addition, acne thrives on inflammation. The ketogenic diet eases and reduces inflammation, thus enabling the body to decrease acne eruptions. Fatty acids, which are found in abundance in fish, are a known anti-inflammatory.

While research is still being done, it seems likely that a keto diet has beneficial effects for clearer, healthier, more glowing skin.

Keto and Anti-Aging

Many diseases are a natural result of the aging process. While there have not been studies done on humans, studies on mice have shown brain cell improvement on a keto diet.

Several studies have shown a positive effect of the keto diet on patients with Alzheimer's disease. What we do know is that a diet filled with good nutrients and antioxidants, low in sugar, high in protein and healthy fats, while low in carbohydrates, enhances our overall health. It protects us from the toxins of a poor diet.

There is also research indicating that using fatty acids for fuel instead of sugar may slow down the aging process, possibly because of the negative effects that sugar has on our overall wellbeing.

In addition, the simple act of eating less and consuming fewer calories is a matter of basic health, as it prevents obesity and its inherent side effects.

So far, studies have been limited. However, considering the powerful positive effects of the ketogenic diet on our health, it is logical to assume this diet will help us grow older in a more natural way while delaying the natural effect of aging. A normal western diet laden with sugars and processed foods are certainly detrimental to warding off the signs of aging.

Keto and Hunger

One of the major reasons diets fail is hunger. People who diet feel hungry and deprived and simply give up. A low carbohydrate diet naturally leaves people feeling full and satisfied. Less hungry means people will actually remain on the diet longer while consuming fewer calories.

Keto and Eyesight

Diabetics are aware that high blood sugar can lead to a higher risk of developing cataracts. Since the keto diet controls sugar levels, it can help retain eyesight and help prevent cataracts. This has been proven in several studies involving diabetic patients.

Keto and Autism

We know the keto diet affects brain functions. In a study on autism, it was found that it also has a positive effect on autism. Thirty autistic children were placed on the keto diet. All showed improved in autistic behavior, especially those on the milder autistic spectrum. While more studies are needed, the results were extremely positive.

CHAPTER 3 – KETO DIET AND CANCER

Cancer has turned into a serious disease in our modern society. While cancer was not a large factor before the 20th century (it did exist, of course), our modern diet and sedentary lifestyle have made cancer the second primary cause of death, with 1600 American dying from this disease every day. It appears that our bodies do not react well to being exposed to daily toxins.

While any cancer treatment must be guided by your physician, it is a good idea to discuss the keto diet and what it can do to help in the treatment of this disease.

A cancer-specific keto diet may consist of as much as 90 percent fat. There is a very good reason for that. What doctors do know is that cancer cells feed off carbohydrates and sugar. This is what helps them grow and multiply in number.

As we have seen, the keto diet dramatically reduces our carbohydrate and sugar consumption as our metabolism is altered. What the keto diet does, in essence, is remove the "food" on which cancer cells feed and starves them. The result is that cancer cells may die, multiply at a slower rate, or decrease.

Another reason why a keto diet is able to slow down the growth of cancer cells is that by reducing calories, cancer cells have less energy to develop and grow in the first place. Insulin also helps cells grow. Since the keto diet lowers insulin level, it slows down the growth of tumorous cells.

When on the keto diet, the body produces ketones. While the body is fueled by ketones, cancerous cells are not. Therefore, a state of ketosis may help reduce the size and growth of cancer cells.

One study monitored the growth of tumors in patients suffering from cancer of the digestive tract. Of those patients who received a high carbohydrate diet, tumors showed a 32.2 percent in growth. Patients on a keto diet showed a 24.3 percent growth in their tumor. The difference is quite significant.

Another study involved five patients who combined chemotherapy with a keto diet. Three of these patient went into remission. Two patients saw a progression of the disease when they went off the keto diet.

More studies are needed, but these numbers are encouraging.

The keto diet may help prevent cancer from occurring in diabetic patients in the first place. People with diabetes have a higher risk level to develop cancer due to elevated blood sugar levels. Since the ketogenic diet is extremely effective at decreasing the levels of blood sugar, it may prevent the initial onset of cancer.

From what research has discovered so far, ketogenic diet may:

1. Stop the growth of cancer cells.
2. Help replace cancerous cells with healthy cells.
3. Change the body's metabolism and enable the body to "starve" cancer cells by depriving them of needed nutrition.
4. By lowering the body's insulin level, the ketogenic body may prevent the onset of cancer cells.

On a ketogenic diet specifically for cancer, your fats should be 75 to 90 percent, protein 15-20 percent, and less than 5 percent carbohydrates.

<u>Foods to Eat</u>

1. Egg, including yolks

2. All green, leafy vegetables, as well as cauliflower, avocado, mushrooms, peppers, cucumbers, and tomatoes.

3. When choosing dairy, opt for full-fat version of cheeses, butter, sour cream, yogurt, and milk.

4. Eat nuts such as walnuts, almonds, filberts, and sunflower and pumpkin seeds.

<u>Foods to Eat in Moderation</u>

1. Have one serving of root vegetables, such as yams, parsnip, carrots, and turnips per day.

2. Fruits contain sugar, so treat them like candy. One small piece per day.

3. A glass of dry wine, vodka, whiskey and brandy once a week. No cocktails with sugars.

4. A small piece of chocolate with 75 percent or higher cocoa content once a week.

<u>Foods to Avoid</u>

1. Any food containing sugar, including cereals; soft drinks, juices, and sports drinks, candies, and chocolate. Limit artificial sweeteners as much as possible.

2. Starchy food such as pasta and potatoes, breads, potato chips, and french fries, cooking oils, and margarine.

3. All beers.

The initial use of the keto diet had nothing to do with weight loss or diabetes management, for which it is now so well-known. Instead, the diet was created by a doctor in 1924 to help his patients suffering from epilepsy.

Epilepsy is a nervous system disorder that can bring on recurrent seizures at any time. The symptoms can be spasms and convulsions, or an unusual psychological view of the world. In any case, it is caused by abnormal brain activity. The severity of the symptoms varies from person to person. A person is diagnosed with epilepsy only if he or she suffers from more than two seizures in one full day. Anyone can suffer from this disorder, but it seems to affect young children the most, perhaps because the young brain is still in a state of development.

Seizures are frequently managed by drugs. Sometimes they work; sometimes, they don't.

As far back as 1924, however, Dr. Russell Wilder of the Mayo Clinic conducted groundbreaking research and created the ketogenic diet to help children suffering from epilepsy. It was remarkably effective, but doctors lost interest when new anti-seizure medications came on the market. It was easier for them to prescribe medication than to discuss diet.

However, people who used the keto diet to treat seizures continued seeing remarkable success. Today, doctors are returning to using the low carbohydrate, high-fat diet to treat their patients. The results have been extremely promising.

In 1998, the Journal of Pediatrics published a study involving 150 children who experienced seizures despite taking popular anti-seizure medications. The children were placed on the ketogenic diet for one year which the researchers assessed their progress.

Eighty-three percent of the subjects were still in the study after 3 months. Over one-third of the children showed a 90 percent decrease in seizures. At the end of the year, slightly more than half of the subjects had remained on the diet, and a quarter of them experienced a 90 percent decrease in seizures. The numbers indicate that the keto diet has a tremendously positive effect on children who suffer from seizures. The researchers consider it more effective than medication in many cases.

For anyone with children who experience seizures, the inclusion of a keto diet in the child's treatment should be discussed with his or her physician.

Another research on the effects of the keto diet on childhood epilepsy involved 145 children. The children were divided into two groups, with one group being treated with medication while the other group receiving a ketogenic diet. Seventy-four percent of the ketogenic diet group were successful in reducing seizures.

There have been more studies of childhood epilepsy and the keto diet. These have sparked new and considerable interest within the medical profession.

Chapter 5 - Keto Diet and Blood Pressure

One-third of American adults suffer from high blood pressure. It is a serious health problem that can lead to heart attacks and strokes. Obviously, the higher the blood pressure, the greater the risk. Aging and obesity greatly increase the chances of developing high blood pressure.

Blood pressure is usually treated with a variety of medications, some of which can have side effects. The best blood pressure is 120/80. High blood pressure is the result of hypertension, and the causes aren't always clear, but we live in an increasingly tense world, and more and more people are dealing with high blood pressure.

It is a known fact that people suffering from high blood pressure frequently carry excess belly fat and can become at risk for type 2 diabetes. To get at the root of all these problems may require a change in lifestyle.

The symptoms of high blood pressure can be caused by an overload of carbohydrates in the diet, more than the body is able to handle. As we've discussed, carbohydrates are converted into sugars, which raise the body's blood sugar level, forcing the body to create additional insulin. Insulin stores fat, and an excess of insulin can lead to obesity. All of this can have a negative effect on your blood pressure.

Consuming fewer carbohydrates decreases both the level of insulin and the blood pressure level. This simple dietary change can make a huge difference in your blood pressure.

In an interesting study released in the Archives of Internal Medicine, 146 overweight people took part in a weight-loss experiment. The people were divided into two groups. One group was put on a ketogenic diet containing a maximum of 20 grams of carbohydrates, while the other group was given the weight-loss drug orlistat, in addition to being counseled to follow a low-fat regimen.

Both groups showed similar weight loss. What surprised the researchers was that half of the keto group showed a decrease in blood pressure, while only 21 percent of the low-fat diet group had any decrease in blood pressure. While weight loss itself would bring about a lowering of blood pressure, the study suggests that a decrease in carbohydrate intake can help lower blood pressure even more.

It was found that potassium specifically had a huge effect on lower hypertension. Doctors recommend at least 4,700 mg of potassium each day for anyone wishing to lower his or her blood pressure.

<u>Foods high in potassium are:</u>

- Avocado

- Acorn squash

- Bananas

- Coconut water

- Dried apricots

- Pomegranate

- Salmon

- Spinach

- Sweet potato

- White beans

While all these foods are permitted on the ketogenic diet, limit your intake of sweet potato and beans, which are starchy and can contain a high level of carbs.

Chapter 6 - What Do I Eat on a Keto Diet?

Some people associate the keto diet with the bad word "fat," and are quick to dismiss it. Nothing could be further from the truth. Fat is allowed, because it is converted into energy. Our body needs healthy fats to thrive. Other foods on the diet could not be healthier. When you're eating ketogenic, you're filling your body with nutrition. Let's take a look at the foods you'll be eating.

As this book has already pointed out, the elimination of processed foods and sugar is one of the best things you can do for your health in general. Processed foods are filled with toxic preservatives that do nothing for you but rob you of your good health. Fresh is always better. When purchasing anything at the market, get into the habit of reading labels. They can be very sneaky and revealing.

Keep your carbohydrates under 50 grams a day, and you'll feel the difference. A stricter ketogenic diet will contain approximately 20 grams of carbs a day.

Food to Eat on a Ketogenic Diet

1. Seafood

Everyone knows about the healthy fatty acids, vitamins and minerals in seafood. Very few of us eat enough. The keto diet encourages the consumption of all things from the sea. Shrimp and crabs are carb-free, and other shellfish contain only a low amount of carbohydrates.

Fatty fish, such as salmon and sardines, are highly recommended because of their high omega-fatty acid content. Fish truly is brainfood. Enjoy at least two servings or more of seafood a week on the keto diet. Simple canned tuna counts as seafood.

2. Vegetables

Can a diet that recommends unlimited green, leafy vegetables be anything but healthy? They are extremely low in carbohydrates and bursting with vitamins, antioxidants, and the fiber we need daily. Green vegetables such as broccoli, spinach, and kale are believed to decrease the risk of heart diseases and cancer. Cauliflower and turnips can be prepared to look and taste like rice or mashed potatoes, with much less starch and carbohydrates.

"Starchy" vegetables, such as potatoes or beets do have carbs and should be limited on the keto diet.

3. Dairy Foods

a. There are cheeses to satisfy everyone's taste. They are high in fat content for energy, high in protein and calcium, and low in carbohydrates.

b. Yogurt and cottage cheese are a great source of protein and calcium. They are low-carb and fit well into the ketogenic lifestyle. Be sure to stick with plain yogurt, as the flavored types contain a lot of sugar, as are the so-called "low fat" versions of yogurt. You can flavor yogurt and cottage cheese yourself with a few berries and nuts.

4. Avocados

Avocados are truly "superfood." They are high in important vitamins and minerals, including potassium. According to a study, avocados are also believed to help lower cholesterol by 22 percent.

Loaded with nutrients and delicious taste, avocados only have 2 grams of net carbohydrates. Use them in salads and sandwiches.

5. Meat and Poultry

The keto diet lets you eat plenty of meat. Meat contains very few carbs and is high in protein to help you build muscles. Whenever possible, choose healthy, grass-fed meats, which are higher in fatty acids.

6. Eggs

Eggs are high in protein and contain a mere 1 gram of carbohydrates. As they are also inexpensive, they are ideal for anyone on a ketogenic diet.

Eggs also make you feel full, thereby helping you eat less. Many people take pride in only consuming the whites of eggs, but the true nutrition lies in the yolk, so be sure to eat the egg in its entirety.

7. Coconut Oil

Too many people are unfamiliar with coconut oil, another "superfood." It is perfect for people dealing with diabetes and has been used with Alzheimer patients.

Coconut oil can be used in most recipes in place of butter or oil. You can also use it for frying and sautéing.

8. Dark Chocolate

Did you know that dark chocolate has a high amount of antioxidants? As a matter of fact, dark chocolate is reaching superfood status. Chocolate with 80 percent or higher real cocoa powder can lower your blood pressure.

An ounce of 80 percent dark chocolate contains 10 grams of carbohydrates, so it definitely counts as a healthy snack. Keep in mind the lower of cocoa content, the less healthy the chocolate will be. Milk chocolate does not count as a healthy chocolate.

Foods to Avoid on a Ketogenic Diet

The keto diet has a lot less restricted foods than many other diets. Sugar, of course, should be avoided. That doesn't mean you can't enjoy sweet desserts. There are many keto-friendly recipes that substitute unsweetened apple sauce for sugar in baked goods. Substitute sweeteners such as Stevia can also be used in moderation.

Keep in mind that fruits are healthful, but they do contain a great deal of sugar, so limit the amount you eat to just a few slices a day. Fruit juices are concentrates that have vitamins but lack fiber. And their sugar content is extremely high. Read the label on any bottle of juice before buying. The best juices are "green" with just a hint of fruit for flavoring.

Be careful with cereals. Most are packed with sugar and robbed of any nutrients. Many claim, "nutrition added," but all that means is that all nutrition has been removed and replaced with a small amount, and a whole lot of sugar for taste. One hundred percent bran cereal will fit into your keto diet, and you can sweeten it with a handful of berries. Just be sure to examine all labels in the cereal aisle. They can be very tricky. Also, remember that honey, too, is considered as sugar.

Totally omit white starches from your diet. They are nothing but empty calories. This includes white bread, pasta, and rice. Buy the wholegrain version, instead, and enjoy in moderation.

Legumes and beans are healthy for you, but they are high in carbohydrates. You can have them occasionally; just make sure you keep it within your daily 20 – 5o carb-gram count.

Alcohols tend to be empty calories, but certain spirits will be better for you than others. Beer is filled with carbs and should be off your keto diet. The expression "beer belly" exists for a reason. Enjoy a glass of wine, instead. Of course, there are variances in different types wine. Dry wines contain a minimum amount of sugar, while sweet dessert wines contain much more.

Pure alcohol such as whiskey and vodka are carb-free, but they do contain calories, so have a care. Mixing alcohol for fancy cocktails usually creates a haven for sugar, so avoid those.

Wine coolers may be a tasty treat, but in reality, they are just sugary sodas with some added alcohol. They should definitely not be on your keto diet at any time.

Chapter 7 - Keto Diet For Rapid Weight Loss

Many people confuse the ketogenic diet with low carb diets or paleo diets. However, there are considerable differences of which you should be aware.

Keto v. Low Carb

A low-carb diet can be anything it wants to be, as long as it is low in carbohydrates. And "low" is rarely defined. On a low-carb diet, you simply make random food choices that curb your carb intake arbitrarily. Since there is no real number, you might still be consuming too many carbs.

Most importantly, what the low-carb diet lacks is that all-critical ketonic state that turns carbs into fats and provides your body with a new and effective source of fuel. This can leave you very hungry and tired.

The ketogenic diet has a specific ratio of carbs to fats to protein. This manipulation is critical, and it's why a low carb diet won't work as well, if at all.

Keto v. Paleo

The Paleo is also a low-carb-type diet. It is based on the assumption that eating the way our cavemen ancestors did, i.e., meat and no carbs, sugars, or grains, is the healthiest type of diet.

There are problems with this reasoning. First, our ancestors never experienced the kind of diseases that we face. The ketogenic diet is specifically a "healing" diet that is meant to benefit the body in many ways and help prevent diseases. The paleo diet does not do that.

Also, the paleo diet is based on eating meat instead of manipulating the ratio of fats, carbohydrates, and protein to achieve a ketonic state that uses fat as fuel.

Ketogenic Diet

Basically, ketogenic is low-carb, but it is much more.

There is a reason the ketogenic diet has become so popular. It helps improve your overall wellbeing in addition to helping you lose weight. You have more energy during the day, and you feel sated and full, thereby reducing the cravings for unhealthy snacks. In essence, you are eating less, but better. That's what makes the keto diet so unique and successful.

The ketogenic diet is not magic pill made up by some gurus. Countless studies and testimonials are able to back the effectiveness of this diet. It is a scientifically proven method that balances your body's fat intake to help achieve optimal weight loss.

By using fat instead of sugar as your primary source of energy, the keto diet induces a state of ketosis, which is achieved when your body stops receiving carbohydrates to turn in glucose. The fewer carbohydrates you consume, the more you force your body to burn fat for energy instead of storing it.

This is why it is possible to lose weight so quickly on the keto diet. It counts carbohydrates instead of calories. Using fats as an additional energy source is what ketosis is all about. It is a natural state that helped our hunter-gatherer ancestors survive in early days.

They feasted on low-carb foods when they could, and fasted when food was scarce. Fat was stored and converted into energy during the scarce times. The ketogenic state is a natural human state, which makes the ketogenic diet so powerful and successful. In addition to the benefits of the keto diet, most people simply enjoy the way it makes them feel better.

Weight loss results on the keto diet differ among individuals, depending on their specific body composition. But weight loss has been the consistent result of people who've been on the keto diet. The keto diet is known as the best weight-loss diet, as well as the healthiest.

A 2017 study divided Crossfit-training subjects into two groups, with both groups following the physical training, but only one group combined the ketogenic diet with the training. The results showed that those on the keto diet decreased their fat mass and weight far more than the other group.

The keto diet group showed an average of 3.5 kilo weight loss, 2.6 percent of body fat, and 2.83 kilos in fat mass, while the other group lost no weight, body fat or fat mass. Both groups showed similar athletic performance ability.

A 2012 study divided overweight children and adolescents into two group; one was put on a keto diet, the other on a low-calorie diet. As in other keto studies, the children on the keto diet decreased their weight, fat mass, and lowered their insulin levels considerably more than the low-calorie group.

Besides more rapid weight loss, a decided advantage of the keto diet over a low-calorie diet is that people actually stick to the keto diet. A low-calorie diet will help you lose weight, but you may be constantly feeling hungry and deprived. That is the main reason most diets fail. Hunger and deprivation are not a part of the ketogenic lifestyle.

Ketosis Explained

As we have stated earlier, the keto diet isn't magic. It is proven science. Ketosis is a natural occurrence that happens when you don't feed your body enough carbohydrates and it is forced to look for energy elsewhere.

You have undoubtedly experienced ketosis when you've missed a meal or have exhausted your body with rigorous exercise. Whenever these things happen, your body helps you out by raising its level of ketones. However, most people eat enough sugar and carbs to keep ketosis from happening.

We love our sugar and carbs, no matter how bad they are for us, and our bodies will happily use them as fuel. And since our bodies

want to help us out, it turns any excess glucose into fat and stores it for future use. Stored fat translated into those ridiculous belly fat that you never want.

The more you restrict your carbohydrate consumption, the more your body will produce ketones. It really has no other options. When we restrict the amount of carbohydrates that we eat, our body will still provide us with energy, but it must turn to another source. And that alternate source is fat that was so thoughtfully stored for emergencies. The result is a state of ketosis. It happens when our body breaks down the fat into fatty acids and glycerol.

Researchers have discovered most of what they know about ketosis from people who fast, thereby depriving them of all sources of energy. After two days of fasting, the body is starting to produce ketones as it breaks down the available protein and begins to use stored fat for fuel. Ketosis is the natural process the body goes through when deprived of other sources of energy.

Obviously, going on a ketogenic diet is healthier than fasting. Ketogenic should become a lifestyle, not a quick weight-loss method. One of the reasons it is so beneficial is that ketones offer protection against diseases and damages that can affect the body.

As mentioned before, keto diet is an excellent tool to prevent many diseases and maintain health and strength longer.

Planning your keto meals will depend largely on your goals. Are you trying to lose weight, or are you on the keto diet to alleviate the symptoms of some disease? The average keto diet will consist of four meals per day, with a total of 100 grams of protein, 25-50 grams of carbohydrates, and 140-160 grams of fat. This can, of course, be adjusted to your personal needs.

For example, if you are on a keto diet to improve cognitive functions, you may want to raise your fat intake to 90 grams a day for optimal results.

Benefits of Intermittent Fasting on Keto

The science behind the ketogenic diet is that the body burns fat when deprived of other sources of fuel. Intermittent fasting is a deliberate deprivation of food and takes the concept a step further. We're not talking long-term fasting.

Intermittent fasting while on a keto diet meant having two meals a day or fasting for one day a week. The fasting time gives the body a chance to rest and rid itself of toxins. It provides an extra boost to the weight-loss benefits of keto and is a great way to jump-start the diet. For weight loss, the keto diet, combined with intermittent fasting, will help you reach your goal faster and easier.

CHAPTER 8 - GETTING STARTED ON THE KETO DIET

You're ready for a new and improved you. Congratulations. There are so many wonderful benefits to the ketogenic diet, you can expect many positive changes, both physical and mental. So, let's not delay and get the journey started.

Clear Your Pantry

We're sure you have plenty of willpower, but there is no need to confront a kitchen filled with tempting sugars and carbohydrates. Make a clean sweep and pack the offending items in a box. Then donate the loot to a needy neighbor or a soup kitchen. They will appreciate your gesture, and you are on your way to a keto lifestyle. If you have family, try to get them involved. If they refuse to refrain from eating carbs and sugar, at least insist they do so away from home. It's a fair request.

Weigh Yourself

The keto diet does not require you to live by the tyranny of the scale. As a matter of fact, as you build up healthy muscles, you might notice a slight initial gain. That's great, so don't worry.

You should, however, have an idea of what your starting point is. If you opted for the keto diet solely to lose weight, you'll be able to track your progress. But don't become a slave to the scale. The occasional weigh-in, perhaps once a week, is enough.

<u>**What About Your Favorite Meals?**</u>

Perhaps the very thought of giving up your favorite foods has prevented you from getting started on the keto way of life. Relax. The truth is, for every dish that you love and can't live without (yes, that includes cheesecake and mashed potatoes!), you can easily find a low-carb substitute that is just as tasty.

First, let's consider items at your market labeled "low carbohydrate." Labels are frustratingly deceiving, and you'd have to be a nutritional expert to understand them. All-too-frequently, off-the-shelf low carb products have simply substituted sugar for carbs, so don't fall for that bit of deceit. You need to learn to read labels with the diligence that you'd read your wealthy uncle's will, but your best bet is to stay away from these products and simply find healthier substitutes. The same goes for anything labeled "low fat," which inevitably means added sugars.

Craving a taco? Use a lettuce wrap instead of a taco shell. Do you want rice or mashed potatoes? Grate or rice a cauliflower, and you won't be able to tell the difference. Can't give up your favorite pasta dish? Turn a zucchini into "zoodles" by slicing it or using a spiral cutter and enjoy your pasta. You absolutely have to have your favorite dessert? On the keto diet, you can. Just bake with almond flour and use unsweetened applesauce and/or avocado to create some sweet smoothness.

Learn about coconut oil, which can be used as a butter substitute in sautéing, frying, and baking. Coconut oil has incredible health benefits, especially for Type-2 diabetics.

On the keto diet, you'll be able to enjoy all your favorite meals, only better.

<u>**Always Stay Hydrated**</u>

The keto diet tends to lower your insulin level, so your kidneys may be excreting more liquid than usual. Be sure to drink plenty of water.

<u>**Condiments Can Be the Enemy**</u>

Don't assume condiments don't count on a diet. On the keto diet, they most certainly do. Ketchup is filled with sugar. Not all salad dressings are equal. Read the label, and never opt for the "fat-free" version. They have merely substituted sugar for fat.

Ordering salads when eating out is one of your best options, but beware of the dressing that the restaurant serves. Either ask about the ingredients, or better, bring your own salad dressing. Don't hesitate to do that, even in a posh eatery where the Maître d' might become spastic at the sight of you pulling salad dressing out of your bag.

Keep Track of Your Ketone Level

It's especially important to remain aware of how your body is responding to the keto diet at the start of the diet. You can do so by doing a simple urine test. You can also purchase a blood ketone meter. It is recommened to perform the test early in the morning.

Friends and Family Can Be Annoying – Bless Their Hearts

Those nearest and dearest to you may not always understand what you are doing. When eating as a group, they may put subtle pressure on you to "just try a bite," or "one slice of cake won't kill you." Or worse, "but I cooked it especially for you!"

It will take resolve to stick to your diet. It may help to fill up on keto-friendly snacks before you sit down and eat. Enjoy some nuts, an avocado, or just a leg of chicken before you eat, and you will be less tempted.

Celebrate!

Celebratory occasions, especially if you're the guest of honor, can be a huge hurdle. When the gang at the office or your parents enter a room with a cake yelling "Surprise!" on your birthday, it's hard to refuse. So, try being a bit sneaky, instead.

By all means gush over the offering. You are expected to do that. You can even help cut slices. Then, discover a sudden and irresistible urge for coffee, which you verbalize loudly and clearly. Gently remove yourself from the center of activity to get coffee for yourself and anyone else. By the time anyone notices, hopefully they've missed the fact that you haven't eaten anything.

Traveling

Traveling while on the keto diet can be a challenge, so be prepared. Pack a personal blender with some avocados and bananas for a few quick and healthful smoothies. Pack some anchovies or tuna for protein.

Eating Out

Eating out isn't as difficult as you may think. Even fast-food places have salads, these days. In any restaurant, stick to meat and vegetables and forego the potatoes and noodles.

You can even navigate the tricky maze in a Chinese restaurant. While abstaining from rice, you can enjoy the following: clear soups, steamed fish with vegetables, egg foo young, stir-fried dishes, Mu Shu without the wrappers are just a few suggestions. Ask your server if your meal can be prepared without cornstarch which is frequently used as a thickener.

Even if you end up in a fast food place that doesn't have salad, simply toss the buns from your burger and just eat the meat. You can do the same at a friend's house or at a BBQ.

Exercise

The keto diet will build muscle mass and give you added energy. Don't forget to incorporate exercise into your daily routine. It can be as simple as walking more, taking the stairs, or joining a gym.

How Long Should You Stay on a Ketogenic Diet"

The amount of time spent on the diet can vary and should be discussed with your doctor. Many people who use the ketogenic diet for weight loss remain on the diet for several weeks, until they have achieved a goal, then they turn to a paleo diet or other maintenance eating. You do not want to lose weight only to return to your old eating habits.

If you are on the ketogenic diet for medical or therapeutic reasons, check with your doctor to ascertain if you should remain on the diet for a longer period of time.

CHAPTER 9 – KETO RECIPES

You can take your favorite recipes and turned them "keto." Below are a few recipes to show you how easy it is. It might be an excellent idea to buy a keto cookbook for your kitchen.

Two of the most important keto recipes are the simple cauliflower rice and "zoodles." They couldn't be easier to prepare. People can get frustrated on the keto diet when they crave pasta and rice. These two recipes definitely satisfy those cravings; they taste just like the real thing. The zoodles can be used for any pasta dish.

(SOUP RECIPES)

KETO BROCCOLI SOUP

Serves:4
Prep Time: 10   Minutes
Cook Time: 30   Minutes
Total Time: 40   Minutes

INGREDIENTS

- olive oil
- 1 cup chicken broth
- 1 cup heavy whipping cream
- 6 oz. shredded cheddar cheese
- salt
- 5-ounces broccoli
- 1 celery stalk
- 1 small carrot
- ½ onion

DIRECTIONS

1.   In a pot add olive oil over medium heat

2.   Add onion, carrot, celery and cook for 2-3 minutes

3.   Add chicken broth and simmer for 4-5 minutes

4.   Stir in broccoli and cream

5.   Sprinkle in cheese and season with salt

KETO TACO SOUP

Serves:8
Prep Time: 10   Minutes
Cook Time: 10   Minutes
Total Time: 20   Minutes

INGREDIENTS

-        2 lbs. ground beef
-        1 onion
-        1 cup heavy whipping cream
-        1 tsp chili powder
-        14 oz. cream cheese
-        1 tsp garlic
-        1 tsp cumin
-        2 10 oz. cans tomatoes
-        16 oz. beef broth

DIRECTIONS

1.   Cook for a couple of minutes, onion, garlic and beef

2.   Add cream cheese and stir until fully melted

3.   Add tomatoes, whipping cream, beef broth, stir and bring to boil

KETO CHICKEN SOUP

Serves:4
Prep Time: 10   Minutes
Cook Time: 30   Minutes
Total Time: 40   Minutes

INGREDIENTS

- 2 boneless chicken breast
- 20-ounces diced tomatoes
- ½ tsp salt
- 1 cup salsa
- 6-ounces cream cheese
- avocado
- 2 tablespoons taco seasoning
- 1 cup chicken broth

DIRECTIONS

1. In a slow cooker place all ingredients and cook for 5-6 hours or until chicken is tender

2. Whisk cream cheese into the broth

3. When ready, remove and serve

KETO SPINACH SOUP

Serves:2
Prep Time: 5   Minutes
Cook Time: 15   Minutes
Total Time: 20   Minutes

INGREDIENTS

- ¼ lbs. spinach
- 2 oz. onion
- ¼ lbs. heavy cream
- ½ oz. garlic
- 1 chicken stock cube
- 1,5 cup water
- 1 tablespoons butter

DIRECTIONS

1. In a saucepan melt the butter and sauté the onion

2. Add garlic, spinach and stock cube and half the water

3. Cook until spinach wilts

4. Pour everything in a blender and blend, add water

5. Serve with pepper and toasted nuts

KETO TOSCANA SOUP

Serves:4
Prep Time: 10   Minutes
Cook Time: 30   Minutes
Total Time: 40   Minutes

INGREDIENTS

- 1 lb. Italian sausage
- ½ cup whipping cream
- 1 tsp garlic
- 2 cup kale leaves
- 1 bag radishes 16-ounces
- 1 onion
- 30-ounces vegetable broth

DIRECTIONS

1. Cut radishes into small chunks and blend until smooth

2. In a pot add onion and sausage, cook until brown, add radishes, broth

3. Cook on medium heat, add heavy whipping cream, kale leaves

4. Cook for a couple minutes

5. Remove and serve

KETO PARMESAN SOUP

Serves:4
Prep Time: 10   Minutes
Cook Time: 30   Minutes
Total Time: 40   Minutes

INGREDIENTS

- 1 broccoli
- 1 tsp pepper
- 1 tablespoon butter
- 1 tablespoon cheese
- 1 onion
- ½ cup warm
- 1 tsp salt
- ½ cup heavy cream

DIRECTIONS

1. In a saucepan add onion and cook

2. Stir in broccoli and cook until soft

3. Combine with heavy cream and place in a blender, blend until smooth

4. Return the soup to the saucepan, season with salt

5. Serve and sprinkle with parmesan

KETO CAULIFLOWER SOUP

Serves:4
Prep Time: 10   Minutes
Cook Time: 30   Minutes
Total Time: 40   Minutes

INGREDIENTS

- ½ head of cauliflower
- ½ cup heavy cream
- ½ red bell pepper
- 1 tsp salt
- 1 tsp pepper
- 1 tablespoon butter
- 1 tablespoons parmesan cheese
- 1 tsp herbs

DIRECTIONS

1. In a saucepan melt butter, add cauliflower and cook until soft

2. Remove from saucepan and set aside

3. Melt butter and sauté and bell pepper

4. In a food processor add cauliflower mixture, pepper and cook for 4-5 minutes

5. Season with salt and pepper

6. Garnish with parmesan and serve

KETO BROCCOLI CHEESE SOUP

Serves:2
Prep Time: 10   Minutes
Cook Time: 20   Minutes
Total Time: 30   Minutes

INGREDIENTS

-       2 cups broccoli
-       3 cups chicken broth
-       1 onion
-       1 cup heavy cream
-       6 oz. cream cheese
-       1 tablespoon hot sauce
-       3 tablespoons butter
-       1 clove garlic
-       6 oz. cheddar cheese

DIRECTIONS

1.   In a saucepan melt butter, add onion, garlic and sauté until soft

2.   Pour in heavy cream, chicken broth, stir in broccoli

3.   Cover and continue cooking for 12-15 minutes

4.   Add cheese and cook until melted

5.   Stir in hot sauce and enjoy

KETO QUESO SOUP

Serves:4
Prep Time: 10   Minutes
Cook Time: 30   Minutes
Total Time: 40   Minutes

INGREDIENTS

- 1 lb. chicken breast
- 1 tablespoon taco seasoning
- 1 tablespoon avocado oil
- 1 can diced green chilies
- 6-ounces cream cheese
- ½ cup heavy cream
- salt
- 2 cups chicken broth

DIRECTIONS

1. In an iron Dutch oven heat oil over medium heat stir in taco seasoning and cook for 1-2 minutes

2. Add broth, chicken and simmer for 20 minutes, remove chicken and shred

3. Stir in cream cheese and heavy cream into the soup, once the cheese has melted, add the chicken back to the soup, season with salt and serve

KETO CRAB SOUP

Serves:6
Prep Time: 10   Minutes
Cook Time: 10   Minutes
Total Time: 20   Minutes

INGREDIENTS

-       1 tablespoon butter
-       1 tablespoon seasoning
-       6-ounces cream cheese
-       ¾ cup parmesan cheese
-       1 lb. lump crabmeat

DIRECTIONS

1.   In a pot melt butter and add seasoning, cream cheese and whisk until smooth

2.   Add parmesan cheese, crab meat and reduce heat

3.   Simmer until is done

4.   Remove and serve

KETO SALAD

Serves:2
Prep Time: 10   Minutes
Cook Time: 10   Minutes
Total Time: 20   Minutes

INGREDIENTS

- 1 slice bacon
- 3-ounces chicken breast
- 1-ounce cheddar cheese
- 1 tablespoon olive oil
- 1 tablespoon apple cider vinegar
- ½ avocado
- 1 head romaine lettuce

DIRECTIONS

1. Chop all ingredients and place them in a bowl

2. Mix well and add pepper, oil and vinegar

KETO BROCCOLI SALAD

Serves:2
Prep Time: 10   Minutes
Cook Time: 10   Minutes
Total Time: 20   Minutes

INGREDIENTS

-        20-ounce raw broccoli
-        1 cup bacon
-        ½ red onion
-        1 cup avocado mayo
-        1 cup macadamia nuts
-        ½ cup Monkfruit sweetener
-        1 tablespoon organic apple cider vinegar

DIRECTIONS

1.   Place Macadamia Nuts in a blender and blend until smooth

2.   Place all ingredients in a bowl and mix well, pour over Macadamia Nuts mixture and
serve

KETO GREEN SPRING SALAD

Serves:4
Prep Time: 10   Minutes
Cook Time: 30   Minutes
Total Time: 40   Minutes

INGREDIENTS

-       2-ounces mixed greens
-       2 tablespoons pine nuts
-       1 tablespoon raspberry vinaigrette
-       1 tablespoon parmesan
-       1 slice bacon
-       salt and pepper

DIRECTIONS

1.   Cook bacon until crispy

2.   Place greens in a bowl with the rest of ingredients

3.   Top with bacon and serve

KETO EGG SALAD

Serves:4
Prep Time: 10   Minutes
Cook Time: 30   Minutes
Total Time: 40   Minutes

INGREDIENTS

- 6 eggs
- 2 celery stalks
- 2 green onion stalks
- 1 green pepper
- 1 tsp mustard
- 2/3 cup mayonnaise

DIRECTIONS

1. Hard boil eggs and remove to a bowl

2. Chop green pepper, onions and celery

3. In a bowl mix all the ingredients and serve

KETO CAESAR SALAD

Serves:4
Prep Time: 10   Minutes
Cook Time: 30   Minutes
Total Time: 40   Minutes

INGREDIENTS

- 10 oz. chicken breasts
- 1 tablespoon olive oil
- salt
- 2 oz. bacon
- 6 oz. romaine lettuce
- 1 oz. parmesan cheese

DRESSING

- ½ cup mayonnaise
- 1 tablespoon chopped filets of anchovies
- 1 garlic clove
- 1 tablespoon mustard
- ½ lemon zest
- 1 tablespoon parmesan cheese

DIRECTIONS

1. In a bowl mix all ingredients for the dressing and set aside

2. Preheat oven to 400 F and place chicken breast in a baking dish and bake for 15-20 minutes

3. In a bowl place sliced chicken, all the salad ingredients, dressing and mix well

4. Serve with parmesan cheese

KETO PEPPERONI SALAD

Serves:4
Prep Time: 10   Minutes
Cook Time: 30   Minutes
Total Time: 40   Minutes

INGREDIENTS

-       ½ avocado
-       12 slices pepperoni
-       1 oz. Mozzarella pears
-       Italian seasoning

DIRECTIONS

1.   In a bowl mix all ingredients and serve

KETO CHICKEN SALAD

Serves:4
Prep Time: 10   Minutes
Cook Time: 30   Minutes
Total Time: 40   Minutes

53

INGREDIENTS

- 2 ribs celery
- ½ tsp pink Himalayan
- 1 tsp fresh dill
- ½ cup pecans
- 1 lb. chicken breast
- ½ cup mayo
- 1 tsp mustard

DIRECTIONS

1. Preheat oven to 425 F and bake chicken breast for 15-20 minutes

2. Remove chicken and cut into small pieces

3. In a bowl mix all ingredients and toss until chicken is fully coated

4. When ready, add dill and serve

KETO TUNA SALAD

Serves:4
Prep Time: 10   Minutes
Cook Time: 30   Minutes
Total Time: 40   Minutes

INGREDIENTS

-     1 can tuna
-     ½ tsp dill
-     1 boiled eg
-     1 slice bacon
-     1 tablespoon mayo
-     1 tablespoon sour cream
-     1 tsp mustard
-     1 tablespoon onion

DIRECTIONS

1. Prepare bacon, onion and boil egg

2. In a bowl place tuna, add egg and onion and the rest of ingredients

2. Top with bacon and serve

SPINACH SALAD

Serves:4
Prep Time: 10   Minutes
Cook Time: 30   Minutes
Total Time: 40   Minutes

INGREDIENTS

- 2 cups spinach
- ½ avocado
- 1 strawberry

DRESSING

- 2 slices bacon
- 1 tablespoon avocado oil
- pinch red pepper flakes
- 1 tsp oregano
- ½ tsp garlic powder
- ½ tsp salt
- half lemon

DIRECTIONS

1. In a bowl mix all dressing ingredients

2. In another bowl mix salad ingredients and pour dressing over

3. Mix well and serve

KETO POTOTO SALAD

Serves:1
Prep Time: 10   Minutes
Cook Time: 10   Minutes
Total Time: 20   Minutes

INGREDIENTS

- 1 cauliflower
- 1 tablespoon mustard
- 1 tsp celery seeds
- ½ tsp salt
- ½ cup celery
- 1 tsp dill
- ½ cup sour cream
- ½ cup mayonnaise
- 2 stalks green onions
- 2 hard boiled eggs
- 1 tablespoon white vinegar

DIRECTIONS

1.   In a bowl prepare dressing by whisking together sour cream, celery seed, salt, mayonnaise, vinegar and mustard

2   In another bowl mix salad ingredient, pour dressing and mix well

KETO MONGOLAIN BEEF

Serves:2
Prep Time: 10   Minutes
Cook Time: 10   Minutes
Total Time: 20   Minutes

INGREDIENTS

- 1 lb. flat iron steak
- ½ cup coconut oil
- 2 green onions

LOW CARB MONGOLIAN BEEF MARINADE

- ½ cup coconut aminos
- 1 tsp ginger
- 1 clove garlic

DIRECTIONS

1. Cut the flat iron steak into thin slices

2. Add the beef to a ziplock bag and add coconut aminos, garlic and ginger, marinate for 1 hour

3. Add coconut oil to a wok and cook beef on high heat for 2-3 minutes

4. Add green onions, cook for another 1-2 minutes

5. Remove and serve

PEPPERONI KETO PIZZA

Serves:2
Prep Time: 10   Minutes
Cook Time: 10   Minutes
Total Time: 20   Minutes

INGREDIENTS

- 1 cauli'flour foods crust
- 2 oz. pepperoni
- ½ cup pizza sauce
- salt
- 2-ounces fresh mozzarella
- ½ cup jalapeno

DIRECTIONS

1. Preheat oven to 375 F and place pizza crust on a vented pizza pan, cook for 8-10 minutes

2. Add mozzarella, sauce, pepperoni and jalapeno

3. Place back in the oven for 5-6 minutes

4. Remove and serve

QUICK KETO PIZZA

Serves:4
Prep Time: 10 Minutes
Cook Time: 10 Minutes
Total Time: 10 Minutes

INGREDIENTS

PIZZA CRUST

- 2 eggs
- 1 tablespoon parmesan cheese
- 1 tablespoon husk powder
- ½ tsp Italian seasoning
- salt
- 2 tsp frying oil

TOPPINGS

- 1 oz. mozzarella cheese
- 2 tablespoons. Tomato sauce
- 1 tablespoon chopped basil

DIRECTIONS

1. In a bowl mix all pizza crust ingredients

2. Spoon the mixture into a pan, cook for 1 minute per side

3. Add cheese, tomato sauce and broil for 1-2 minutes until cheese is bubbling

MUSHROOMS PIZZA

Serves:2
Prep Time: 10   Minutes
Cook Time: 15   Minutes
Total Time: 25   Minutes

INGREDIENTS

- ¼ cup rao's marinara
- pepperoni
- sliced baby bella mushrooms
- sliced ripe olives
- mozzarella

DIRECTIONS

1. Preheat oven to 375 F

2. Spray a pie plate with a non-stick cooking spray

3. Spread marinara on bottom of pie plate

4. Layer mushrooms, pepperoni, olives and top with mozzarella

5. Bake for 10 minutes and serve

BUFFALO KETO CHICKEN TENDERS

Serves:2
Prep Time: 10   Minutes
Cook Time: 30   Minutes
Total Time: 40   Minutes

INGREDIENTS

-       1 lb. chicken breast tenders
-       1 cup almond flour
-       1 egg
-       1 tablespoon heavy whipping cream
-       5 oz. buffalo sauce
-       salt

DIRECTIONS

1.   Preheat oven to 325 F

2.   Season chicken with salt, pepper and almond flour

3.   Beat 1 egg with heavy cream

4.   Dip each tender in the egg and then into seasoned almond flour

5.   Place tenders on a baking sheet and bake for 25 minutes or until crispy

6.   Remove and serve

KETO LASAGNA

Serves:4
Prep Time: 10   Minutes
Cook Time: 30   Minutes
Total Time: 40   Minutes

INGREDIENTS

-       1 lb. ground beef
-       1 cup sauce
-       ¾ cup mozzarella
-       6 tablespoons ricotta
-       salt, onion powder, Italian seasoning

DIRECTIONS

1.   Preheat oven to 350 F, brown beef and season

2.   Being to layer a deep dish with noodle, ricotta, sauce mix and sprinkle with mozzarella, top with cheese

3.   Bake for 20-25 minutes

4.   Remove and serve

KETO PARMESAN CASSEROLE

Serves:3
Prep Time: 10   Minutes
Cook Time: 30   Minutes
Total Time: 40   Minutes

INGREDIENTS

- 2 cups cooked chicken
- ½ tsp basil
- 1 slice bacon
- ½ cup marinara sauce
- ½ tsp red pepper flakes
- ¾ cup mozzarella cheese
- ½ cup Parmesan cheese

DIRECTIONS

1.   Preheat the oven to 325 F

2.   Lay out the chicken in the pan and spread the marinara sauce all over

3.   Dredge the top with parmesan, red pepper flakes, mozzarella and sprinkle bacon and basil

4.   Bake for 20-25 minutes, remove and serve

KETO CHEESE MEATBALLS

Serves:2
Prep Time: 10   Minutes
Cook Time: 10   Minutes
Total Time: 20   Minutes

INGREDIENTS

-       ½ lbs. beef mince
-       2 tablespoons parmesan cheese
-       ½ tsp salt
-       ½ tsp pepper
-       ¼ lbs. cheese
-       1 tsp garlic powder

DIRECTIONS

1.   Cut the cheese into cubes

2.   Mix all dry ingredients with the ground beef

3.   Wrap the cubes of cheese in mince and pan fry the meatballs

KETO CHEESY BACON CHICKEN

Serves:4
Prep Time: 10 Minutes
Cook Time: 30 Minutes
Total Time: 40 Minutes

INGREDIENTS

- 5 chicken breasts
- 2 tablespoons seasoning rub
- ½ lbs. bacon
- 3 oz. shredded cheddar
- barbecue sauce

DIRECTIONS

1. Preheat oven to 375 F and spray a baking sheet with cooking spray

2. Rub both sides of chicken breast with seasoning rub and top with bacon, bake for 25 minutes

3. Remove from oven, sprinkle with cheese and serve

KETO CHEESEBURGER

Serves:2
Prep Time: 10   Minutes
Cook Time: 60   Minutes
Total Time: 70   Minutes

INGREDIENTS

-        2 lbs. ground beef
-        2 eggs
-        ½ cup grated parmesan
-        1 small onion
-        1 tsp salt
-        1 tsp garlic powder
-        ½ cup cheddar cheese

DIRECTIONS

1.   In a bowl mix all ingredients except cheddar cheese, add the end add cheese cubes

2.   Place mixture into a sprayed oven dish and form a meatloaf shape

3.   Bake at 325 F for 50 minutes

4.   Remove and serve

(CAKE)

CHEESECAKE KETO FAT BOMBS

Serves:12
Prep Time: 10   Minutes
Cook Time: 10   Minutes
Total Time: 20   Minutes

INGREDIENTS

- 5 oz. cream cheese
- 2 oz. frozen strawberries
- 2 oz. butter
- 1 oz. swerve sweetener
- 1 tsp vanilla extract

DIRECTIONS

1. Puree the strawberries using a blender

2. In a bowl mix sweetener, vanilla, pureed strawberries and mix well

3. Microwave cream cheese and combine with the rest of ingredients

4. Add butter to the mixture and mix with an electric mixer

5. Divide into 10-12 round silicone molds and freeze for 1-2 hours before serving

KETO BROWNIES

Serves:12
Prep Time: 10   Minutes
Cook Time: 20   Minutes
Total Time: 30   Minutes

INGREDIENTS

-        ½ cup almond flour
-        ½ tsp baking powder
-        1 tablespoon instant coffee
-        2 oz. chocolate
-        1 egg
-        ½ tsp vanilla extract
-        ½ cup cacao powder
-        2/3 cup Erythritol
-        8 tablespoons utter

DIRECTIONS

1.   Preheat oven to 325 F

2.   In a medium bowl whisk almond flour, baking powder, Erythritol, cocoa powder and instant coffee

3.   In another bowl melt chocolate and butter and whisk in the eggs and vanilla

4.   Add to dry ingredients and mix well

5.   Transfer batter into baking dish and bake for 20 minutes

6.   Remove and serve

KETO ICE CREAM

Serves:2
Prep Time: 10 Minutes
Cook Time: 20 Minutes
Total Time: 30 Minutes

69

INGREDIENTS

- 2 cups heavy cream
- 1 tablespoon milk powder
- ½ tsp xanthum gum
- 1 tsp vanilla extract
- 1 cup whole milk
- ½ cup truvia baking blend

DIRECTIONS

1. In a bowl mix milk powder, sweetener, xanthum gum

2. Pour in cream, vanilla extract, milk and mix until sweetener is dissolved

3. Pour into ice cream maker and churn until set

4. Serve when ready

KETO EGG CREPES

Serves:2
Prep Time: 10   Minutes
Cook Time: 10   Minutes
Total Time: 20   Minutes

INGREDIENTS

-       5 eggs
-       5 oz. cream cheese
-       1 tsp cinnamon
-       1 tablespoon sugar substitute
-       butter

FILLING

-       7 tablespoons butter
-       ½ cup sugar substitute
-       1 tablespoon cinnamon

DIRECTIONS

1.   Blend all of the crepe ingredients until smooth

2.   Pour batter into the pan and cook 1-2 minutes per side

3.   Remove and pour mixture over the crepes

4.   For crepes mixture mix cinnamon and sweetener in a bowl

5.   Serve when ready

KETO NAAN

Serves:4
Prep Time: 10   Minutes
Cook Time: 30   Minutes
Total Time: 40   Minutes

INGREDIENTS

- ½ cup coconut flour
- 1 tablespoon psyllium husk
- 1 tablespoon ghee
- ½ tsp baking powder
- ½ tsp salt
- 1 cup boiling water

DIRECTIONS

1. In a bowl mix all ingredients and refrigerate

2. Divine the dough into 6 balls

3. Heat a cast iron skillet over medium heat and place ice naan ball

4. Cook for 2-3 minutes remove and serve

PEANUT BUTTER COOKIES

Serves:12
Prep Time: 10   Minutes
Cook Time: 30   Minutes
Total Time: 40   Minutes

INGREDIENTS

- 1 cup peanut butter
- 1 tsp vanilla
- 1 tsp baking powder
- ½ tsp salt
- ½ cup keto sweetener
- 1 egg

DIRECTIONS

1. Preheat oven to 325 F

2. Cream together all ingredients

3. Refrigerate for 15-20 minutes

4. Roll dough into balls and place on a parchment paper

5. Bake for 12-15 minutes

BUTTERY KETO CREPES

Serves:2
Prep Time: 10   Minutes
Cook Time: 10   Minutes
Total Time: 20   Minutes

INGREDIENTS

- 3 eggs
- ½ tsp vanilla extract
- ½ tsp cinnamon
- 3 oz. cream cheese
- 2 tsp sweetener
- 2 tablespoons butter

DIRECTIONS

1. In a blender place all the ingredients and blend until smooth

2. In a skillet pour batter and cook each crepe for 1-2 minutes per side or until ready

3. Remove and serve with berries, maple syrup or jam

KETO LEMON FAT BOMB

Serves:4
Prep Time: 10   Minutes
Cook Time: 10   Minutes
Total Time: 20   Minutes

INGREDIENTS

-        ½ cup coconut oil
-        3 tablespoons butter
-        3 oz. cream cheese
-        2 tsp lemon juice
-        2 tsp sugar substitute

DIRECTIONS

1.   Place all ingredients in a mixing bowl and mix thoroughly

2.   Spoon 2 tablespoons into cupcake holders and freeze

3.   Remove and serve

PEANUT BUTTER BALLS

Serves:4
Prep Time: 10   Minutes
Cook Time: 30   Minutes
Total Time: 40   Minutes

75

INGREDIENTS

- 1 cup peanuts finely chopped
- 1 cup peanut butter
- 1 cup powdered sweetener
- 6 oz. sugar free chocolate chips

DIRECTIONS

1.   In a bowl mix peanut butter, sweetener, chopped peanuts, divide dough into 12 pieces and shape into balls and place on a wax paper

2.   Melt chocolate and dip each peanut butter ball in the chocolate and place back on the wax paper

3.   Refrigerate and serve

NUT FREE KETO BROWNIE

Serves:8
Prep Time: 10   Minutes
Cook Time: 20   Minutes
Total Time: 30   Minutes

INGREDIENTS

- 5 eggs
- ¼ lb. butter
- 2 oz. cocoa
- ½ tsp baking powder
- 2 tsp vanilla
- ¼ lb. cream cheese
- 3 tablespoons sweetener of choice

DIRECTIONS

1. Place all the ingredients in a lender and blend until smooth

2. Pour mixture into a baking dish

3. Bake at 325 F for 20 minutes

4. Remove slice into squares and serve

COFFEE SMOOTHIE

Serves:1
Prep Time: 5   Minutes
Cook Time: 5   Minutes
Total Time: 10   Minutes

INGREDIENTS

- 5 oz. cold coffee
- 3 oz. heavy cream
- 3 oz. almond milk
- 1 oz. sugar free chocolate syrup
- 1 oz. caramel syrup
- 1 tablespoon cocoa
- 12 oz. ice

DIRECTIONS

1. In a blender place all the ingredients and blend until smooth

2. Pour in a glass and serve

CHAI PUMPKIN SMOOTHIE

Serves:1
Prep Time: 5   Minutes
Cook Time: 5   Minutes
Total Time: 10   Minutes

INGREDIENTS

- ¾ cup coconut milk
- 2 tablespoon pumpkin puree
- 1 tablespoon MCT oil
- 1 tsp chai tea
- 1 tsp alcohol free vanilla
- ½ tsp pumpkin pie spice
- ½ frozen avocado

DIRECTIONS

1. In a blender place all the ingredients and blend until smooth

2. Pour in a glass and serve

CASHEW SMOOTHIE

Serves:1
Prep Time: 5   Minutes
Cook Time: 5   Minutes
Total Time: 10   Minutes

INGREDIENTS

-       1 cup cashew mik
-       1 tablespoon keto MCT oil
-       1 tablespoon keto nut butter
-       1 tsp maca powder
-       1 handful ice

DIRECTIONS

1.   In a blender place all the ingredients and blend until smooth

2.   Pour in a glass and serve

BREAKFAST SMOOTHIE

Serves: 1
Prep Time: 5   Minutes
Cook Time: 5   Minutes
Total Time: 10   Minutes

INGREDIENTS

-        ½ cup almond milk
-        ½ cup coconut milk
-        ½ coconut yoghurt
-        ½ tsp stevia
-        3 strawberries

DIRECTIONS

1.   In a blender place all the ingredients and blend until smooth

2.   Pour in a glass and serve

KETO MILKSHAKE SMOOTHIE

Serves:1
Prep Time: 5   Minutes
Cook Time: 5   Minutes
Total Time: 10   Minutes

INGREDIENTS

- 6 oz. plain almond milk
- 3 oz. crushed ice
- 1 oz. heavy whipping cream
- 1 oz. raspberries
- ¾ oz. sweetener of choice
- ½ oz. cream cheese

DIRECTIONS

1. In a blender place all the ingredients and blend until smooth

2. Pour in a glass and serve

AVOCADO SMOOTHIE

Serves:1
Prep Time: 5   Minutes
Cook Time: 5   Minutes
Total Time: 10   Minutes

INGREDIENTS

-       ½ avocado
-       2 tablespoons cocoa powder
-       2/3 cup coconut milk
-       ½ cup crushed ice
-       ½ cup water
-       pinch of salt
-       1 tsp lime juice
-       stevia

DIRECTIONS

1.   In a blender place all the ingredients and blend until smooth

2.   Pour in a glass and serve

COLLAGEN SMOOTHIE

Serves:1
Prep Time: 5   Minutes
Cook Time: 5   Minutes
Total Time: 10   Minutes

83

INGREDIENTS

-        4 ice cubes
-        ½ avocado
-        1 scoop keto chocolate collagen
-        1 tablespoon chia seeds
-        1 tablespoon almond butter
-        ¾ cup heavy whipping cream
-        1 cup water

DIRECTIONS

1.   In a blender place all the ingredients and blend until smooth

2.   Pour in a glass and serve

FAT BOMB SMOOTHIE

Serves:1
Prep Time: 5   Minutes
Cook Time: 5   Minutes
Total Time: 10   Minutes

INGREDIENTS

-       2.5 oz avocado
-       1 scoop collagen
-       1 tablespoon cacao powder
-       1 cup almond milk
-       1 cup ice

DIRECTIONS

1.   In a blender place all the ingredients and blend until smooth

2.   Pour in a glass and serve

CINNAMON SMOOTHIE

Serves:1
Prep Time: 5   Minutes
Cook Time: 5   Minutes
Total Time: 10   Minutes

INGREDIENTS

- ½ cup coconut milk
- ½ cup water
- 2 ice cubes
- 1 tablespoon coconut oil
- ½ tsp cinnamon
- 1 tablespoon chia seeds
- ½ cup vanilla protein powder

DIRECTIONS

1. In a blender place all the ingredients and blend until smooth

2. Pour in a glass and serve

TROPICAL SMOOTHIE

Serves:1
Prep Time: 5   Minutes
Cook Time: 5   Minutes
Total Time: 10   Minutes

INGREDIENTS

-        ½ tsp banana extract
-        ½ tsp blueberry extract
-        ½ tsp mango extract
-        stevia
-        1 tablespoon oil
-        ½ cup sour cream
-        ice cubes
-        ¾ cup coconut milk

DIRECTIONS

1.   In a blender place all the ingredients and blend until smooth

2.   Pour in a glass and serve

The Mediterranean Diet

CHAPTER 1

THE MEDITERRANEAN DIET: ITS RICH HISTORY IS AN

AMALGAMATION OF CULTURES

The first thing you may be wondering is how in the world did the Mediterranean Diet come about? The Mediterranean Diet, also called the Greek Mediterranean Diet, came about after researchers looked at the dietary habits of the Crete people. A plethora of studies revealed its ability to boost longevity and reduce the possibility of suffering from Alzheimer's disease.

Many historians call this region of the world "the Cradle of Society." Why? Within the geographical borders, a whole history of the ancient world occurred. Along the region was the Nile River as well as two well-known basins – the Euphrates and Tigris. The civilizations of this region included the Babylonians, Assyrians, Persians, and Sumerians.

It wasn't too long that the Cretans rose to power, and not long after, the Phoenicians and Greeks came to power. It permitted the territory to become a good land between the West and East. It allowed the people to become one in the Mediterranean, bringing together cultures, languages, religions, customs and various thought processes.

Region's Power Struggle Changes Course Of The Mediterranean Diet

And, it all changed the history of how the Mediterranean Diet came to be because their eating habits merged. What's known is that the Mediterranean Diet includes oil products, wine, and bread (as noted by the Greek culture) and the strong preference for sheep cheese, fish, seafood, vegetables (as noted by the Roman culture).

The rich class consumed fresh fish, either grilled or fried in olive oil, and seafood such as oysters, eating them fried or raw. Roman slaves were provided with less quality food such as bread and olives and olive oil each month. They rarely had any meat but would sometimes be given salted fish.

It wasn't long before this Roman tradition clashed with the Germanic way of life and food, especially for nomads who lived within the forest. They would hunt, farm and gather for their food, using pig fat to cook in the kitchen. The grains that were grown were not for bread making but beer making.

These two cultures clashed and led to the partial amalgamation of eating habits. It was, however, the Roman culture of the Mediterranean style that would not waver. The primary elements of this diet were wine and triad oil bread, which were exported to various parts of the European continent.

The important elements in Christian mass were bread, wine, and oil, but they were soon adopted to feed everybody in the European region. This new food culture was the result of the union of two very different cultures – Germanic and Roman Empire. And, it eventually made passage into a third – the Arab world, which had its own distinct food culture on the southern Mediterranean shores.

Muslims increased the importance of agriculture, which swayed the food model to bring plant species that only the wealthy social classes had known – rice, sugar cane, spices, spinach, eggplant, citrus, etc.

The Islamic culture played an integral part in changing the Mediterranean diet that the Romans had first established and offered a new culinary model to it. There are a plethora of foods – recipes and traditions - Muslims added to the diet.

The Mediterranean Diet underwent more changes after the Europeans discovered America. The change is the result of the purchase of new items – corn, chili, potatoes, peppers, tomatoes and various types of beans. Europeans saw the tomato has an exotic curiosity – an ornate fruit that was edible – that would eventually become the Mediterranean diet's staple.

If vegetables are the main component of the Mediterranean Diet, it's important to understand how important cereals played in the diet. For poor classes, cereals gave them a chance to feel full. Of course, the kinds of cereals they consumed were based on geographical location and traditions of the people who lived in the Mediterranean region. Bread, couscous, pasta, paella, polenta and soups were various methods used to eat cereals.

As you see, the Mediterranean diet underwent a plethora of changes, from region to region, and the diet people know today is due to the introduction of various foods of those different regions.

What Is The Mediterranean Diet Then

The diet is a food model that boosts the safety and quality of food and where they first originated. The cuisine is simple but loaded with tastes and imagination that allows anyone to take advantage of every aspect of the diet. Preservation of the customs and traditions of the

Mediterranean Basin people is seen as an ethical choice.

Food has a profound effect on people's health, and good nutrition is necessary to stave off various metabolic diseases like hypertension, diabetes, and obesity. The diet allows for the "sustainable development" of all countries that reside along the Mediterranean border – from the cultural and economic effect food has on the area and its capacity to motivate the local community.

Ancel Keys brought the pattern to the public eye with his "Seven Countries" study, which was published in 1970. It was a landmark study, which looked at the residents of the Mediterranean area and noted they had the lowest amount of coronary heart disease in the world.

Special Note:
While the Mediterranean Diet is known as a diet, it's really not a diet. It doesn't recommend reducing your calorie consumption or eliminating foods that many mainstream American diets suggest. Instead, the diet is all about eating nourishing foods and living an active life.

Chapter 2

What Does The Mediterranean Diet Consist Of

In Chapter 1, you learned how the Mediterranean Diet came about. As you read earlier, it's not an actual diet but a way of life – eating and physical activity – with foods that come from France, Greece, Spain, Southern Italy and other Mediterranean Sea bordering countries. These countries are well-known for consuming foods like fish, fruits, beans, vegetables, whole grains, olive oil, and nuts. They also don't consume a lot of sweets, meats, and cheese.

In fact, they eat more fiber, omega-3 fatty acids, and monounsaturated fats.
The diet is all about heart-health and, because of that, 30 to 40 percent of the diet is healthy fat. Many other diets recommend less than 30 percent for fat consumption. Many of the fats in the Mediterranean Diet are from unsaturated oils like olive oil, fish oil, seed oil and some nut oil (almonds, hazelnuts, walnuts, flaxseed, soybean and canola oil). These oils have a protective element on the heart.

The Mediterranean Diet Pyramid

The Mediterranean Diet Pyramid is a nutrition guide that was developed by Oldways, the Harvard School of Public Health, and the World Health Organization in 1993. It summarizes the Mediterranean Diet pattern of eating, suggesting the types and frequency of foods that should be enjoyed every day.

The pyramid, structured in light of current nutrition research and representing a healthy Mediterranean diet, is based on the dietary patterns of Crete, Greece and southern Italy circa 1960 at a time when the rates of chronic disease were among the lowest in the world, and adult life expectancy was among the highest, even though medical services were limited.

The main concepts of the Food Pyramid are the "proportionality", that is the right amount of foods to choose from for each group, the "portion" standard quantity of food in grams, which is assumed as the unit of measurement to be a balanced feeding, the "variety", i.e., the importance of changing the choices within a food group, and "moderation" in the consumption of certain foods, such as fat or sweets.

As you can see, at the base of the pyramid are grains, followed by fruits and vegetables, legumes, olive oil, low-fat cheese and yogurt, which should be eaten daily. Meat is not excluded, but is given the preference to that of chicken, rabbit and turkey than beef. Along with fish and eggs should be eaten a few times a week, for the supply of high quality protein. Beef or red meat should be eaten a few times a month.

How To Successfully and Easily Incorporate The Mediterranean Diet Into Your Life

Now that you know what the myths and facts are about the Mediterranean Diet, you may be wondering how you can easily incorporate it into your current lifestyle. What changes will you need to make in your dietary plan to add the diet to it? Chances are you've eaten the same way for years, and you may think that changing your diet is going to be difficult.

However, it doesn't need to be.

If you feel it'll be hard to do the Mediterranean Diet, make small steps into the diet. Don't go "balls to the walls" with it, throwing out all the food that doesn't go along with it. Instead, make slow and steady changes – changes that can take place over a couple of weeks to a month.

What Foods Does The Diet Exclude

Before you can know what foods you can have in the diet, it's important you first understand the foods that you shouldn't have in the diet. These foods include:

· Added Sugars – This means no ice cream, candy, table sugar, soda, etc.
· Trans Fats – This is fat found in margarine and many processed foods
· Processed Meat – No hot dogs, sausage, bacon, ham, etc.
· Refined Grains – refined wheat pasta, white bread, etc.
· Refined Oils – No cottonseed oil, soybean oil, vegetable oil, etc.
· Highly-Processed Foods – Don't consume anything that's labeled diet or low-fat (these foods are made in factories)

What Foods Should You Add To Your Diet

Greek Yogurt

This food is great to reduce your hunger pangs and make you feel full. It can also stabilize your blood sugar levels and decrease your cravings. The extra protein in Greek yogurt helps to keep you from overeating. With your body burning more calories, it can digest the protein better than it can with carbs. Yogurt is also great because it has probiotics (good bacteria) that make it easier for you to lose weight.

Beans

Beans contain both insoluble and soluble fiber, and there's no other food that can say that. Soluble fiber will dissolve along with liquid in the stomach to create a viscous gel – this expands so that you feel fuller and hold onto food for a longer period of time. With the insoluble fiber, the liquid is absorbed and gives your digestive system bulk. It works alongside the soluble fiber, so you stay fuller for longer.

Vegetables

It's important to get a good source of micronutrients into your body to ensure it stays active and healthy. According to research, a body that feels tired and fatigued is likely to eat more junk food. Vegetables are necessary to rev up the metabolism and give the body fuel to function. Since vegetables tend to have 90 percent water, it helps stave off dehydration. Dehydration can cause the body to slow the body's metabolism down.

Seafood

99% of Americans don't consume enough omega-3 fatty acids, which is extremely important since it can affect how the body burns fat. The kinds of foods that have omega-3 fatty acids in them include tuna and shellfish. By eating these foods two times a week, you can boost your metabolism-burning power by nearly 400 calories per day. It will also help to keep the fat cells from expanding, especially in the stomach region.

Whole Grains

Whole grains are important in your weight loss efforts. They're loaded with fiber and take more time for you to chew. They boost the saliva juices and will cause the stomach to distend. Whole grains are digested and absorbed slowly, which means a gradual increase in your blood sugar levels – all of which make you feel fuller for a longer period of time. One such food to consider eating is oatmeal.

Herbs & Spices

If you want to speed up your metabolism and lose weight a little faster, add some spice and herbs to your foods. For instance, you can add chili pepper seasoning, hot peppers, nutmeg or cinnamon. These foods will help speed up the metabolism and help you to feel fuller longer.

They ensure you don't eat as much at mealtimes.

Olive Oil

Olive oil has healthy monounsaturated fats than any other oil or food. According to various studies, people who consume olive oil will increase how much energy the body uses at rest. This means while you sleep or sit, your body is burning extra calories. A German study noted that the olive oil scent helped people to feel fuller and eat less money. People who participated in the study ate yogurt that had an olive oil scent extract didn't eat as much and stable blood sugar levels.

And, speaking of olive oils!

Not All Olive Oils Are The Same...

It can be a little overwhelming to go to the store and realize that there's more than one good of olive oil to buy. You must be wondering what kind of olive oil is right for you. Well, here's a closer look at each style:

Extra-Virgin Olive Oil – This is the result of pressing olives and has less than 0.8% acidity. It's got a delicious taste to it. There's no refined oil, making it the healthiest olive oil. It's also the best for your salads.

Virgin Olive Oil – There's no refinement done with this type of olive oil, and it has a higher acidity level – one to four percent. This allows some of the natural flavors and aromas to be retained.

Pure Olive Oil – This is the kind of oil that's seen more often than not in the supermarket. It's a lower-quality refined olive oil, which can differ based on the blend and brand. This is the kind people will use for cooking.

Olive Pomace Oil – This is a solvent-extracted olive oil – extremely cheap and low-grade quality. It's not ideal for consumption, but for cooking.

How Do You Choose The Right Olive To Use

· It's always good to use products with the term extra virgin olive oil, but it's important not to take it for granted.
· Although an oil says it's produced in Italy that doesn't make it Italian.
· The oil will degrade if the time from harvest to processing is long.
· Learn what the harvest date is. Olive oil is good for two years so long as it's stored under ideal conditions – room temperature, dark room. If there's no harvest date on a bottle, don't buy it.

· Smell and taste the oil when you get home. You don't want odors that smell like manure, sweaty socks, old peanut butter or wax.

· Go with dark-glass enclosed olive oil since the dark color will prevent the oil from oxidation and cause rapid deterioration.

· Pick oil for its quality, not color. Olive oils will vary in their color range – light golden color to dark green. This doesn't dictate quality.

· Be mindful of blended oils since they tend to include cheaper, non-olive oils. While not bad, it's not pure olive oil.

· Olive oil is best when used within 18 months. Make sure to use it by the use-by-date.

CHAPTER 3

WHAT ARE THE BENEFITS BEHIND THE MEDITERRANEAN DIET?

Remember, the Mediterranean Diet is loaded with grains, vegetables, fruits, beans, and peas. The diet consists of very little meat, and the majority of the fat is the result of eating nuts or using olive oil. There have been many studies looking at the health benefits of the Mediterranean Diet, and those studies found that it decreased the risk for many obesity related diseases. What are some of the benefits that are associated with Mediterranean Diet?

6 Primary Benefits Of The Mediterranean Diet

Reduced Consumption Of Sugar and Processed Foods

The Mediterranean Diet is all about natural or as near natural to nature foods such as fruits, vegetables, peas, beans, olive oil and minute amounts of animal products. It's not like the American diet, which is loaded with GMOs and artificial ingredients such as high fructose corn syrup, flavor enhancers, and preservatives. People who follow the Mediterranean Diet consume more fruit and minute amounts of homemade desserts that contain nature sugars like honey.

Fish, like anchovies and sardines, is a major staple of this diet along with moderate amounts of yogurt and sheep, goat or cow cheeses. These foods are not typically seen in Western diets. Does this mean people who follow the Mediterranean Diet are vegetarians? Not at all! It just means they don't consume as much meat or food. They go with healthier, lighter foods. And, all of this can lower your cholesterol levels, improve your heart health and boost your omega-3 fatty acid intake. Plus, it will help with weight loss.

You Drop The Weight In A Healthy Manner

If you want to lose weight and not feel hungry – to keep the weight off – the Mediterranean Diet is a sustainable method that promotes weight loss. You decrease your amount of fat intake and increase your consumption of nutrient-rich foods.

When it comes to this diet, how you do it is up to you. If you want to reduce your carb consumption, you can do so. If you want to consume more protein than carbs, you can do that too. Your body needs healthy fatty acids, which will help you control any weight gain, make you feel full and control your blood sugar level. Plus, you'll feel more energetic and have a better mood.

Boost Your Heart Health

A traditional Mediterranean diet has a plethora of omega-3 and monounsaturated fats foods, which can reduce your chance of developing heart disease. Research has shown that olive oil is loaded with alpha-linolenic acid, which can reduce the cardiac death risk by 30 percent and unexpected cardiac death by 45 percent. People who consume more olive oil had a better blood pressure rate than people who consumed other kinds of oils such as sunflower, vegetable, etc.

It Can Help Prevent Cancer

Plant foods – vegetables and fruits – are a major part of the Mediterranean diet, and these foods help to fight cancer. They provide your body with antioxidants, protect DNA from being damaged, reduce the possibility of cell mutation, reduce inflammation and slow down or prevent tumor growth. Olive oil is also beneficial in preventing cancer development, especially bowel and colon cancers.

Reduce The Chance For Diabetes Development

Various evidence notes that the diet can help with anti-inflammatory issues, reducing the chances of the body developing chronic inflammation, type 2 diabetes, and metabolic syndrome. It can prevent diabetes by controlling the extra insulin (hormone controlling blood sugar levels and leads to weight gain).

With blood sugar levels regulated and eating better types of carbs and proteins, your body will burn fat more effectively. The American Heart Association notes the Mediterranean diet is much higher in fat, but that it's healthier fat. Remember, the diet is 40 percent carbohydrates, 20 to 30 percent quality proteins and 30 to 40 percent healthy fats. The diet is low in sugar, getting most of it from fruit and locally made desserts.

Reduce Stress Levels and Relax

One of the biggest reasons to consider this diet over many of the others is the relaxing feeling you get from it. With inflammation reduced, you can spend your time cooking a healthy meal at home and get a good night's rest. You can also spend your time outside, surrounding yourself with nature and people you love.

You know how detrimental chronic stress can be – how bad it is for your health and weight. With a slow-down lifestyle like you'd see with the Mediterranean Diet, you can choose foods that are healthier for you and partake in physical activity as well. All of this can help you to relieve your stress level and feel happier overall.

As you see, there are so many benefits the Mediterranean diet has to offer. And, the research behind the diet supports every one of them. Researchers carried out a study that looked at the diet and its effects on cardiovascular disease. The participants were noted to have a high cardiovascular risk; those who followed the diet reduced their chances for a cardiovascular problem by 30 percent.

Who Can Use The Mediterranean Diet?

Anybody who wants to eat healthy, feel better and lose weight can follow the Mediterranean Diet. It can fit into one anyone's lifestyle including a child's. Plus, children who have been introduced to a healthy diet and exercise are far more likely to keep up the lifestyle when they become adults.

CHAPTER 4

DON'T BELIEVE THE DIET MYTHS

In chapter 3, you learned what the benefits were to the Mediterranean Diet. However, you can
only experience those benefits by ensuring you successful follow the diet. This means you must understand what the myths are behind the Mediterranean Diet. With so much misinformation out there about the diet, it's no wonder people assume the diet doesn't work. Know the facts, and realize it's not a lose weight quick method.

Myth 1 – It Takes A Plethora Of Money To Follow The Diet
The truth of the matter is less expensive than other diets (Atkins, Weight Watchers, and South Beach) because your meals are being created from lentils, beans or peas, which are a primary source of protein. The other diets promote processed or prepackaged foods that are loaded with sodium, cholesterol, and other unhealthy ingredients.

Myth 2 – You Eat A Lot Of Bread and Pasta
Actually, the Mediterranean people do not consume a large bowl of pasta like Americans do. They keep it as a side dish – ½ cup to 1-cup of serving size.

Myth 3 – You'll Lose Weight If You Do The Traditional Mediterranean Diet Method
People who live on the Greek islands get their good cardiovascular health by being active – walking the steep hills and looking after their animals and garden. It's not just about what you eat, but how active you are in your life. Physical activity is an important part of the diet's success.

Myth 4 – The Diet Is Just About Food
While food plays a role in the diet, it's not the end all, be all to the diet's success. Remember, you must be physically active too.

Myth 5 – Every Vegetable Oil Is The Same and Good For You

If it were that simple, then there would be no problems, right? The reality is that there are two kinds of unsaturated vegetable oils – traditional, cold-pressed oils like peanut oil and extra virgin olive oil are loaded with monounsaturated fats and are well-ingrained in the Mediterranean Diet. These kinds of oils are developed without using heat or chemicals to extract them.

Myth 6 – Avoid All Alcohols

Actually, research has found that wine – red wine specifically – is beneficial to people who follow the Mediterranean Diet. Of course, it's all about moderation – less than five ounces for women and less than 10 ounces for men. If you have any kind of drinking problem or there's a history of alcohol abuse in the family, it may be best to avoid alcohol.

Myth 7 – You Can Consume All The Cheese You'd Like

One of the biggest myths is that you can consume all the cheese you want – something people of the Mediterranean region will eat. However, you cannot eat all you want since it will lead to unwanted calories and it has saturated fats. If you want to eat cheese, you must do so in moderation. Consider eating goat or feta cheese to get the flavor you want without a lot of the cheese.

Myth 8 – There's No Reason To Work Out

It's true that most people living in the Mediterranean region 50 years go didn't exercise at the gym, but they did participate in physical activity such as manual labor and walking instead of driving. If you want to go to the gym, go for it.

Myth 9 – The Diet Is Loaded With Fats

The kind of fats that are permitted in the Mediterranean Diet are monounsaturated fats such as the various types of olive oil. People automatically (and wrongly) assume that the presence of olive oil makes it a bad choice for diets. Olive oil is loaded with good cholesterol and decreases the body's cholesterol.

Myth 10 – You Don't Eat As Much Food

Many people think the Mediterranean Diet decrease how much food you consume. The reality is that the lifestyle encourages people to eat healthy, which can reduce their calorie intake. It encourages them to add more fruits and vegetables in their diet rather than high-calorie drinks and foods.

Epilogue

Remember, this diet isn't really a diet but a lifestyle change, which means you don't have to make significant changes to your lifestyle. You don't have to count calories, which is something your body should be dealing with. Your body knows what amount of calories it needs and what it'll do with those calories.

There's no reason to weigh yourself every day because body weight will vary. On top of that, you could actually gain weight or maintain it but lose fat (thanks to strength training). Along with ignoring the calorie counting, you need to avoid complex calculations such as the ever-disgusting Body Mass Index (BMI). BMI is not the best way to determine if you're overweight or obese. Someone who is "big-boned" will weigh more, but that doesn't mean they have fat.

Is the Mediterranean Diet something you should be doing for yourself? Research has shown that the diet (more like a lifestyle change) is one of the healthiest you can partake in. If you want to lose weight, it's a diet that should be something you continue doing for at least six months – but it would be better if it were for good. Watch how much you eat, what you eat and maintain a healthy exercise program.

As noted in an earlier chapter, there are so many ways this diet is good for your body. Remember, it's good for your heart, it reduces your cholesterol levels and blood pressure, decreasing your chance of suffering from heart disease. You are less likely to be diagnosed with type 2 diabetes because your diet is focused more on fruits, not refined sugars and carbs. It also helps to prevent certain kinds of cancers such as bowel cancer.

Is the Mediterranean Diet something you should incorporate into your life?

If you want a diet that you can see yourself doing for the rest of your life, this is the diet for you. You don't have to forgo all the good things you already have in your diet, but add healthier foods and partake in different exercises to see its benefits. It's a really a very flexible diet – that anyone of any age – young and old – can get involved in.

But before we proceed with our meal plan and

recipes...

What are the main fundamentals of cooking and baking?
Cooking and baking have both evolved over time, and still differences can be observed from country to country.

However, all great bakers and chefs abide by the following:

1. **Baking is precision, cooking is art.**

Two rules naturally follow:

a. Measure, measure, measure (baking): Any minor changes in a recipe - too much flour, overmixing egg whites - can make the difference between perfect colored macarons and cracked, unleavened shells.

First of all the right tools will make cooking or baking a pleasure. Avoid plastic kitchen utensils as they are often made with toxic plastic chemicals. I prefer to use stainless steel measuring cups and spoons which are made by KUFL.

- Made of premium grade stainless steel
- US measurements are molded directly into the handle along with liquid equivalents & metric conversions (milliliters)... even if you're an expert converter, it still very convenient!
- Heavy-duty and built to last

You can easily find any of these wonderful sets by searching Amazon.com for "kufl measuring cups" or "kufl measuring spoons" or just use this link. (I will get a small reward if you purchase it through my link.)

b. Always taste as you go (cooking). Ingredients change with the season and terroir, and may carry more or less at a given time of the year. Likewise, the heat in chilies and peppers vary greatly, so you can not take anything for granted.

2. A dish is only as good as the ingredients that compose it
In his Guide to Modern Cookery, August Escoffier said that:
"The choice of the raw material is a matter of demanding vast experience on the part of the chef; for the old French adage which says that "La sauce fait" should not be in the slightest degree inferior to its accompanying sauce. "

Two principles naturally follow:

a. Use quality ingredients

Cooking and baking are the combination and transformation of different ingredients to improve the desirability, taste, and digestibility of food. Even with the greatest amount of technique and creativity, it is ultimately your production.

b. Know how to choose your ingredients

Ingredient selection is a crucial step in culinary. Escoffier, again, advised against "entrusting the choice of kitchen provisions for people unacquainted with the profession, and who, never having used the goods, they have to buy, are able to judge only very superficially of their quality or real value, and can not form any estimate of their probable worth after the cooking process. "

Good news is, it is a skill that can be developed through experience cooking and eating. The more you eat apples, the more discerning and capable you will be to choose good apples (or at least apples that you like). Touch, sight, and smell are your best asset to select your ingredients.

3. Each ingredient has a role to play

a. In baking, each ingredient has a particular chemical and structural function, and you can do it properly, you can not, you can not properly substitute an ingredient from a given recipe or even successfully create your own recipes.

Generally, the flour provides the structure; baking powder and baking soda help the dough to rise while giving the cake a delicate, airy texture. Eggs act as a connector, binding the ingredients together; butter and oil soften. Sugar adds sweetness and gives your final product a denser, shiner finish. Milk or water deliver moisture.

b. Cooking is the perfect balance of the five basic flavors: sweet, salt, bitter, sour and umami.

Your best bet is to train your tongue to detect the various tastes and correct accordingly. In doing so, keep in mind that salt does more than make food taste salty. It enhances sweetness and suppresses bitterness.Water to dilute your dish will lift it out of its intensity.

Beware taste saturation. The more you taste the food. So punctuate your sampling with palate-cleansing glugs of water.

4. Never waste ingredients

Chefs are the most important of the cost of goods, and food is the ultimate sin in a professional kitchen. Concretely, that means giving a second life to dishes (e.g. cooking with leftovers) or scraping the bottom of your bowl to find that last drop of batter.

7 Day Mediterranean Meal Plan

(Mediterranean Diet Recipes)

Meal Day 1

Breakfast: Classic Eggs Florentine – 270 calories
Snack: Crostini with Tomato and Mozzarella – 380 calories
Lunch: Stuffed Shells with Spinach and Cheese – 439 calories
Snack: Mediterranean Salad with Figs and Mozzarella – 286 calories
Dinner: Tuna Noodles with Artichokes and Olives – 422 calories

Calories Total Day 1: 1802 calories

Classic Eggs Florentine

Category: Breakfast
Difficulty: Easy
Servings: 2
Nutrition facts per serving: 270 calories

Ingredient List:
Extra virgin olive oil
2 slices of prosciutto
2 room temperature eggs
1 large tomatoes in 1-inch thick slices
2,5 ounces of small spinach leaves (approximately 2,5 cups)
1/4 cup diced onion
1,5 cloves minced garlic
1/3 cup grated Pecorino
Romano cheese
1,5 tbsp olive oil
0,4 cup heavy cream
1/2 tbsp lemon juice
1/8 tsp ground nutmeg
1/2 tbsp salt
Ground black pepper to taste

Instructions:
Over preheat temperature: 400 degrees Fahrenheit.
Position a rack in the middle of the oven. Prepare a flat baking sheet by spraying it with non-stick cooking spray made with vegetable oil. Lay the slices of prosciutto out flat on the baking sheet. Place this in the oven for 6 to 8 minutes until the meat is crisp. Remove the prosciutto when cooled and crumble it into a bowl.

Creamy Spinach Mixture
Set a stove burner to medium-high and place a skillet on it. Pour the olive oil in and wait a moment for it to heat up. Add the onion and cook for approximately 5 minutes until all pieces are soft. Then, add the garlic and cook for 30 seconds until the pungent aroma is released. Next, add all of the spinach leaves and nutmeg. Cook about 1 to 2 minutes until the spinach wilts. Pour the heavy cream over the spinach mixture and wait for it to simmer gently. Cook for approximately 5 minutes, stirring several times until it thickens. Turn off the stove burner and remove the pan. Mix in the grated cheese and stir well. Add salt and pepper according to personal taste preferences.

Poached Eggs

Bring 1,5 inches of water, 1/2 tbsp of salt and 1/2 tbsp of lemon juice to a simmer in a deep saucepan. Carefully crack an egg into the water. This can be done directly or done into a small bowl first and then introduce the egg to the hot water. Stir the simmering water with a wooden spoon so it swirls gently around the egg. Allow the egg to cook for 2 to 3 minutes so the white is set but the yolk has not cooked all the way through. Poach each egg separately. Use a slotted spoon to scoop each egg from the water and drain on a clean paper towel.

Presentation and Serving

Position each thick tomato slice on a small plate. Add salt and pepper to taste. Top this with a quarter of the spinach mixture. Then, add a poached egg on top. Use the cooked and crumbled prosciutto for additional flavor and garnish. Serve right away before the Eggs Florentine cools.

Crostini with Tomato and Mozzarella

Category: Appetizers
Difficulty: Easy,
Servings: 4
Nutrition facts per serving: 385 Calories,
Fat - 18.4g
Carbs - 35.9g
Protein - 17.6g
Cholesterol - 45mg
Sodium - 453mg

Ingredient List:
1/2 French baguette
1,5 tbsp extra virgin olive oil
2 cloves garlic, halved
3 plum tomatoes, seeded and chopped
1/2 bunch fresh basil, julienned
1/2 pound fresh mozzarella, sliced

Instructions:
1. Cut baguette into diagonal ½ inch slices for serving.
Brush a light layer of all of oil on each. Toast these in the oven with the broiler on for 2-3 minutes until they are slightly brown. When done, rub a peeled garlic clove over each.
2. Mix together the chopped tomatoes and olive oil. Add in pepper and salt if desired.
3. Arrange the slices of bread on a platter. Add a thin slice of mozzarella, a spoon of the tomato mixture, and a fresh basil leaf to serve.

Stuffed Shells with Spinach and Cheese

Category: Lunch
Difficulty: Easy
Servings: 2
Nutrition facts per serving: 439 Calories
Fat - 13g
Saturated Fat - 6g
Fiber - 7g
Carbohydrates - 58g
Protein - 25g,
Folate - 441mcg
Cholesterol - 31mg
Sugars - 9g
Sodium - 569mg

Ingredient List:
8 jumbo pasta shells
1/2 tsp extra-virgin olive oil
2/3 onions, finely chopped
2/3 lbs fresh spinach, trimmed and washed
2/3 cups part-skim ricotta cheese
1/4 cup plain dry breadcrumbs
1/6 cup freshly grated
Parmesan cheese, divided
1/8 tsp ground nutmeg
Salt and freshly ground pepper, to taste
1/3 large egg white, lightly beaten
1 cups prepared marinara sauce, preferably low sodium

Instructions:
1. Preheat oven to 325°F.
2. In boiling water, cook the pasta shells as directed on the package. It should take approximately 15 minutes and the shells should be al dente when they are done. Run under cool water and set them aside for later use.
3. Using medium-high heat on the stovetop, sauté onions in a small amount of oil until they are soft but not browned.
4. Gently stir the spinach in the frying pan until all the leaves are wilted. Pour off the excess liquid when you are done.
5. Stir together the parmesan and ricotta cheeses, breadcrumbs, and nutmeg. Mix the rest of the spinach into this mixture and add the egg white. Blend thoroughly.

6. Use approximately 2 tbsp of the spinach-cheese mix in each pasta shell. Pour 1/2 cup tomato sauce in the 9x13 casserole dish. Spread the shells out to cover the sauce without overlapping each other. Pour the other 1 cups of sauce over everything and add a dusting of parmesan cheese on top.

7. Bake for about 30 minutes until everything is cooked all the way through and the top is browning nicely. A loose sheet of foil can prevent the top from becoming too brown before everything is cooked. Remove from the oven and let the dish rest for 10 minutes before enjoying.

Mediterranean Salad with Figs and Mozzarella

Category: Salads
Difficulty: Easy
Servings: 2
Nutrition facts per serving: 280 calories
Fat - 23g
Saturated Fat - 6g
Carbs - 11g
Sugars - 9g
Fibre - 3g
Protein - 10g

Ingredient List:
100g fine green bean, trimmed
3 small fig, quartered
1/2 shallot, thinly sliced
65g ball mozzarella, drained and ripped into chunks
25g hazelnut, toasted and chopped small handful basil leaves, torn
1,5 tbsp balsamic vinegar
1/2 tbsp fig jam or relish
1,5 tbsp extra-virgin olive oil

Instructions:
1. Blanch the green beans in hot water with salt for 3-4 minutes. Drain them and pat dry with paper towels or allow to dry in a colander. When dry, pour them out on a platter or large plate.
2. Arrange fig quarters, shallot slices, chunk cheese, chopped hazelnuts, and shredded basil leaves on top of the beans.
3. Combine vinegar, fig jam, and oil with salt and pepper to taste. Blend well and serve over the salad.

Tuna Noodles with Artichokes and Olives

Category: Dinner
Difficulty: Easy
Servings: 2
Nutrition facts per serving: 422 Calories
Fat - 17g
Saturated Fat - 2 g
Fiber - 9g
Carbohydrates - 42g
Protein - 22g
Folate - 126mcg
Cholesterol - 22mg
Sugars - 4g
Sodium - 503mg

Ingredient List:
4 oz tuna steak, cut into thirds
1/8 cup green olives, chopped
1,5 cloves garlic, minced
1 cups grape tomatoes, halved
1/4 cup white wine
1 tbsp lemon juice
3 oz whole-wheat gobbetti, rotini or penne pasta
1 5-oz package frozen artichoke hearts, thawed and squeezed dry
2 tbsp extra-virgin olive oil, divided
1 tsp freshly grated lemon zest
1 tsp chopped fresh rosemary or 1 teaspoon dried, divided
Salt, freshly ground pepper to taste
1/8 cup chopped fresh basil or parsley for garnish

Instructions:
1. Using an outdoor grill or a grilling pan on your stovetop, set it at a medium-high heat. Also, boil a large pot filled with water.
2. Mix the chunks of tuna fish with 1 tbsp of the olive oil, rosemary, salt and pepper, and lemon zest. Grill this for approximately 2-3 minutes on the top, and then turn it over to grill for the same amount of time from the bottom. The tuna should be almost but not quite cooked all the way through.
3. Allow the tuna to cool and then flake it into a small chunks.
4. Cook the pasta in the boiling pot of water, drain it when it is tender, and set it aside.

5. Over medium heat, stir fry the artichoke hearts, garlic, olives, and the rest of the rosemary in the remaining tbsps. of oil. Keep mixing until the garlic browns slightly, which should take 2-4 minutes.

6. Pour in the wine and the tomatoes. Increase the burner temperature and bring this mixture to a boil for a short period of time. The tomatoes should break down somewhat and the liquid quantity should reduce.

7. Add the tuna, pasta, lemon juice, and additional salt or freshly ground black pepper. Mix together well and serve hot with a parsley or basil garnish.

Meal Day 2

Breakfast: Pumpkin pie oatmeal – 280 calories
Snack: Sicilian-style tuna carpaccio – 303 calories
Lunch: Classic Chicken Tetrazzini – 288 calories
Snack: Vegetarian Taco Salad – 392 calories
Dinner: Health-Conscious Carbonara – 493 calories

Calories Total Day 2: 1756 calories

Pumpkin pie oatmeal

Category: Breakfast
Difficulty: Easy
Servings: 2
Nutrition facts per serving: 288 Calories
Total Fat - 13.6g
Saturated Fat - 1.4g
Trans Fat - 0g
Cholesterol - 0mg
Sodium – 74.1mg
Total Carbohydrate – 38.5g
Dietary Fiber – 5.1g
Sugars – 16g
Protein - 5.6g

Ingredient List:
1/2 cup of rolled old fashioned oats
1 cup of almond milk
1/8 cup of pumpkin puree
1/4 tsp of vanilla extract
1/4 tsp of ground cinnamon
1/8 tsp of ground nutmeg
1/4 cup of chopped pecans
1/8 cup of maple syrup

Instructions:
1. Use a small sauce pan to mix oats and milk while heating moderately.
2. Reduce the heat and simmer when it starts to boil. Keep stirring frequently for 3-5 minutes till you observe the required consistency.
3. Add pumpkin puree, vanilla extract, ground cinnamon and ground nutmeg and heat it for a minute.
4. Enjoy the oatmeal after garnishing it with maple syrup

Sicilian-style tuna carpaccio

Category: Appetizers
Difficulty: Easy
Servings: 2
Nutrition facts per serving: 303 Calories
Fat - 19.9g
Saturated Fat - 3.4g
Protein - 24.7g
Carbs - 1.6g
Sugars - 0.8g,
Salt - 0.4g
Fibre - 0.3g

Ingredient List:
2 tbsp capers
4 tbsp rosé wine
1 long fresh red chili
1 x 200 g yellowfin tuna steak
1 lemon
½ bunch of fresh basil
½ bunch of fresh dill
1 small garlic clove extra virgin olive oil rocket leaves, to serve

Instructions:
1. Soak the capers in the rosé wine for approximately 10 minutes.
2. Roast the chili or hold it over the gas flame on your stovetop for approximately five minutes until its skin is black and blistered. Allow this to cool in a bowl, covered with plastic wrap for approximately 10 minutes.
3. Trim the tuna and cut off thin slices against the grain of the meat. Pour or sprinkle ½ lemon's worth of juice over the fish. The juice's acid content will begin the cooking process.
4. Chop the basil, dill, and garlic into fine mince. Remove the capers from the wine and chop those also. Combine these ingredients with olive oil and set aside.
5. Retrieve the cool chili pepper and peel or scrape off the black outer layer. Cut it in half, cut out the seeds, and chop three quarters of it into the bowl with the garlic, herbs, and capers. Stir these together.
6. Lay the tuna slices out in an attractive pattern on a serving dish. Pour a small amount of olive oil over the top, and then later on the chili, caper, and herb mixture.
7. Serve with roasted chili garnish, lemon wedges, and rocket leaves.

Classic Chicken Tetrazzini

Category: Lunch
Difficulty: Easy
Servings: 2
Nutrition facts per serving: 288 Calories
Fat - 6g
Saturated Fat - 2g
Fiber - 3g
Carbohydrates - 35g
Protein - 24g
Folate - 48mcg
Cholesterol - 45mg
Sugars - 5g
Sodium - 551mg

Ingredient List:
2 oz spinach fettuccine
2/3 tsp canola oil
1 leek, white parts only, finely chopped
2 oz button mushrooms, quartered
1/3 tsp chopped fresh rosemary, divided
1 tbsp all-purpose flour
1 cups reduced-sodium chicken broth
1/6 cup low-fat milk
2/3 cups cooked chicken breast, cubed
Grated zest of 1/3 lemon
Lemon juice, to taste
Salt and freshly ground pepper, to taste
25g freshly grated Parmesan cheese
20g fine dry breadcrumbs
1/3 tbsp finely chopped fresh parsley

Instructions:
1. Preheat oven to 425°F. Use non-stick cooking spray on a 3-quart casserole dish.
2. Use the directions to cook the pasta for about 8-10 minutes in boiling water. You want it to be tender yet firm, or al dente, instead of too soft. Drain the fettucine, rinse with cold water, and set to the side for later.
3. Cook the leeks in an oiled skillet using medium temperature setting. They will brown in about 6-8 minutes. Stir in the mushroom pieces and ½ of the rosemary. Five more minutes

will finish the mushrooms and the leeks together. Toss in the flour and stir well. Then, pour in milk
and broth and bring the entire thing to a boil. Cook for about 3-4 minutes until it thickens some.

4. Mix the chopped chicken into the above mixture when it is taken off the stovetop burner. Mix in the cooked pasta as well.

5. Transfer everything to the prepared casserole dish. Top with breadcrumbs, parmesan cheese, parsley, rosemary, and lemon zest. Add salt and pepper as desired.

6. Bake for 25-30 minutes until the edges bubble and the top browns slightly. Let the dish rest for 5-10 minutes before you serve it.

Vegetarian Taco Salad

Category: Salads
Difficulty: Easy
Servings: 6
Nutrition facts per serving: 392 calories
Fat - 16g
Saturated Fat - 5g
Fiber - 9g
Carbohydrates - 52g
Protein - 14g
Folate - 87mcg
Cholesterol - 20mg
Sugars - 10g
Sodium - 481mg

Ingredient List:
2 tbsp extra-virgin olive oil
1 large onion, chopped
1,5 cups fresh corn kernels
(See Note) or frozen, thawed
4 large tomatoes
1,5 cups cooked long-grain brown rice (See Note)
1 15-ounce can black, kidney or pinto beans, rinsed
1 tbsp chili powder
1,5 tsp dried oregano, divided
1/4 tsp salt
1/2 cup chopped fresh cilantro
1/3 cup salsa
2 cups iceberg or romaine lettuce, shredded
1 cup shredded pepper Jack cheese
2,5 cups tortilla chips, crumbled
Lime wedges for garnish

Instructions:
1. Over medium setting on the stovetop burner, heat up a small quantity of oil in a nonstick frying pan. Sauté corn and onions until they start to turn a golden brown. Add a single chopped tomato and the rice, beans, and seasoning. Cook for approximately 5 minutes.
2. Cut up the other tomatoes into bite-sized chunks. Mix these with the salsa, half the oregano, and cilantro in a separate bowl.
3. Combine shredded lettuce with the mixture of rice, beans,

and tomatoes, and ½ the available quantity of salsa. Add in 2/3 cup of the shredded jack cheese.

4. Serve the salad with lime, shredded cheese, salsa, and tortilla chip crumbles on top.

Note: Cut kernels off of corn cobs by standing the ear on one end and using a sharp knife very carefully.

Note: Cook the rice prior to making this recipe. For every ½ cup of rice, pour in 1 cup of water. Bring this to a boil, turn the heat down to a low simmer, and put the lid on the pot until the rice is tender. This should take approximately 45 minutes. Let the rice stand for up to 10 minutes before using in this recipe or serving separately.

Health-Conscious Carbonara

Category: Dinner
Difficulty: Easy
Servings: 2
Nutrition facts per serving: 493 Calories
Fat - 16.4g
Saturated Fat - 5.2g
Protein - 27g
Carbs - 63.6g
Sugars - 9.2g
Fibre - 11.5g

Ingredient List:
200 g fresh or frozen peas
1 tbsp flaked almonds
1 small clove of garlic
½ a bunch of fresh basil
15 g Parmesan cheese
1 lemon
150 g whole wheat spaghetti
1 rasher of smoked bacon
olive oil
1 large free-range egg
100 g fat-free natural yoghurt

Instructions:
1. Boil a pot full of water to cook the pasta in. Before adding the pasta, pour the peas into a colander and dunk them in the boiling water for 25-30 seconds. Put the peas to the side for later. Then, cook the pasta according to the package directions.
2. Over medium heat, toast the almonds in a dry pan. Grind them up smoothly in a food processor at high speeds. Add the garlic, basil, parmesan cheese, salt, and lemon juice to the almonds and continue to blend them together. Finally, add the blanched peas and blend them in until a rough texture forms. You do not want a smooth puree necessarily.
3. Fry small pieces of the bacon in a hot pan. When they are crisp, let them drain on a paper towel of kitchen parchment to get rid of the excess grease.
4. Place ¾ of the blended peas and almond mix into the pan and heat it up.
5. Blend the egg with the yogurt until it is smooth.
6. Put the cooked pasta in the pan with the pea mixture. Allow the pan to cool before adding the egg and yogurt. If the pan or its contents are still hot when you put the egg in, you will

end up with scrambled eggs instead of a smooth and creamy sauce. Mix everything together well.

7. Serve the pasta on a plate with a dollop of the remaining pea mixture on top. Sprinkle with bacon pieces and season with salt and ground pepper to taste. This healthy dish will impress you with its layers of delicious tastes.

Meal Day 3

Breakfast: Banana Bread Waffels – 437 calories
Snack: Panzanella Salad – 307 calories
Lunch: Fettucine with Salmon and Tomatoes – 350 calories
Snack: Tomato carpaccio – 175 calories
Dinner: Chipotle chicken tacos with pineapple salsa – 392 calories

Calories Total Day 3: 1661 calories

Banana Bread Waffels

Category: Breakfast
Difficulty: Easy
Servings: 5
Nutrition facts per serving (1 waffle): 437 Calories
Fat - 18.6
Carbs - 54.75
Fiber - 6.5
Sugar – 8
Protein – 12

Ingredient List:
2 cups all-purpose flour
2 tbsp sugar
1 tsp baking powder
½ tsp baking soda
½ tsp salt
¼ tsp ground cinnamon
Pinch of nutmeg
1 cup milk
2 ripe bananas, mashed
2 large eggs
¼ cup vegetable oil
1 tsp vanilla extract
¼ cup walnuts, chopped

Instructions:
1. Mix together all the dry ingredients: flour, sugar, baking powder and soda, salt, and spices.
2. Use a separate bowl to combine the wet ingredients: milk, eggs, oil, bananas, and vanilla.
3. Combine the contents of each bowl and stir until they are smooth. Add the chopped nuts.
4. Use an electric waffle maker with this batter according to the manufacturer's how-to directions.
5. Serve the banana bread waffles with whipped cream, syrup, sliced fruit, and additional nuts.

Panzanella Salad

Category: Salads
Difficulty: Easy
Servings: 2
Nutrition facts per serving: 307 calories
Fat - 21.7g
Carbs - 22.2g
Protein - 6.6g
Cholesterol - 12mg
Sodium - 551mg

Ingredient List:
1,5 cups day-old Italian bread, torn into bite-size chunks
1,5 tbsp olive oil salt and pepper to taste
1 clove garlic, minced
1 tbsp olive oil
1/2 tbsp balsamic vinegar
1 medium ripe tomatoes, cutinto wedges
1/5 cup red onion, sliced
2-3 basil leaves, shredded
1/8 cup green olives, pitted and halved
1/4 cup fresh mozzarella, cut
into bite-size pieces

Instructions:
1. Preheat oven to 400°F.
2. Combine bread chunks with 1,5 tbsp oil, pepper, salt, and garlic. Spread it on one layer on a baking tray and cook it in the oven until toasted to a golden brown. This should take about 5-10 minutes.
3. Mix together bread, tomato chunks, onion, olives, cheese, and basil.
4. Blend 1 tbsp olive oil with balsamic vinegar. Drizzle this over the bread and other ingredients to serve. Allow approximately 20 minutes for the dish to sit and flavors to incorporate before eating

Fettucine with Salmon and Tomatoes

Category: Lunch
Difficulty: Easy
Servings: 2
Nutrition facts per serving: 350 Calories
Protein - 21g
Carbohydrates - 49g
Sugars - 7g
Fat - 8g
Saturated Fat - 2g
Fibre - 4g
Sodium - 131mg

Ingredient List:
4 oz fettuccine
1tsp extra virgin olive oil
1 tsp garlic, chopped
1,5 cups tomato, chopped
4 oz salmon, canned in water
1 tsp dill weed, dried
1/8 cup parmesan cheese
1/8 cup milk, fat-free

Instructions:
1. Prepare the pasta with the instructions on the package in a boiling pot of water. Drain the cooked fettuccine well and set aside in a covered bowl.
2. Over medium-high heat, combine oil with garlic. Fry this for 1-2 minutes until it browns lightly. Pour in the chopped tomatoes and cook these together. Add all other ingredients and heat them up in the same pan.
3. Combine the tomato and salmon mixture with the pasta and serve right away while everything is still hot.

Tomato carpaccio

Category: Appetizers
Difficulty: Easy
Servings: 2
Nutrition facts per serving: 175 Calories
Fat - 13.4g
Saturated Fat - 6.5g
Protein - 8.5g
Carbs - 3.8g
Sugars - 3.8g

Ingredient List:
3 ripe heirloom tomatoes, sliced
Extra-virgin olive oil
30 g raspberries
80 g burrata, or good quality mozzarella, torn
1/3 bunch small basil leaves
Raspberry vinegar

Instructions:
1. Lay the slices of tomato on an attractive plate.
2. Sprinkle on fresh ground pepper, salt, and olive oil to taste.
3. Smash the raspberries in a bowl with a fork. Add a splash of raspberry vinegar.
4. Arrange torn burrata or mozzarella over the tomatoes and top with raspberry mixture and fresh basil.

Chipotle chicken tacos with pineapple salsa

Category: Dinner
Difficulty: Easy
Servings: 2
Nutrition facts per serving: 392 Calories
Fat - 13g
Saturatet Fat - 3g
Carbs - 37g
Sugars - 21g
Fibre - 5g
Protein -30g

Ingredient List:
250g skinless boneless chicken thighs
1/2 tbsp vegetable oil
1/2 medium onion, chopped
1 tsp sweet smoked paprika
1 tsp ground cumin
1 tbsp cider vinegar
1/2 tbsp chipotle paste
100 ml passata
1 tbsp soft brown sugar
1/4 small fresh pineapple,
cored and chopped
1/4 small pack coriander, chopped
Corn or flour tortillas
Hot sauce to taste

Instructions:
1. Blend chicken thigh meat in a food processor or cut into small chunks with a knife.
2. Combine chicken and ½ the amount of chopped onions in a frying pan with the vegetable oil. Cook until all the meat is browned and crumbled.
3. Sprinkle in all seasonings, vinegar, passata, chipotle, and sugar. Keep cooking and stirring for 5 minutes until the flavors combine evenly.
4. Stir together the other ½ of the chopped onion, pineapple, and coriander. Serve the chicken and salsa with tortillas and other seasonings to taste.

Meal Day 4

Breakfast: Personal-Size Frittata (10 Frittatas) – 220 calories
Snack: Hot Meatball Sandwiches – 456 calories
Lunch: Cioppino – 318 calories
Snack: Spinach Salad with Walnuts and Goat Cheese – 226 calories
Dinner: Salsa spaghetti – 414 calories

Calories Total Day 4: 1634 calories

Personal-Size Frittata (10 Frittatas)

Category: Breakfast
Difficulty: Easy
Servings: 20
Nutrition facts per serving (1 Frittata): 22 calories
Sugar - 0g
Protein - 2g
Carbohydrates - 0.5g
Sodium- 68 ml
Cholesterol - 44 ml
Saturated Fat – 0.5g
Total Fat- 1.5g.

Ingredient List:
Extra virgin olive oil
4 large eggs
2 oz. ham, sliced thin and chopped
1/6 cup Parmesan cheese, grated
1/4 cup whole milk
1 tbsp Italian parsley, chopped
1/4 tsp ground black pepper
1/8 tsp salt

Instructions:
Oven preheat temperature: 375 degrees Fahrenheit.
Use a whisk to combine the eggs, whole milk, salt and pepper in a bowl until they are blended thoroughly. Mix in ham, Parmesan, and Italian parsley.
Coat miniature muffin tin with a total of 24 cups with the vegetable oil cooking spray. Pour the prepared mixture into each until they are filled very close to the brim.
Bake in the preheated oven for approximately 8 to 10 minutes. The frittata should puff up and the egg should be just set in the middle.
Use a rubber or silicone spatula to remove the frittata and place them on a platter or directly onto plates. Serve right away while they are still hot.

Hot Meatball Sandwiches

Category: Appetizers
Difficulty: Easy
Servings: 12
Nutrition facts per serving: 456 Calories
Fat - 23.3g
Saturated Fat - 8.1g
Protein - 25.9g
Carbs - 38.8g
Sugars - 6g
Fibre - 1.7g

Ingredient List:
100 g ciabatta bread
80 g mortadella
4 cloves of garlic, peeled
½ bunch of fresh flat-leaf parsley leaves
400 g lean ground beef
400 g lean ground pork
2 large eggs
30 g Parmesan cheese, freshly grated sea salt freshly ground black pepper
olive oil
1 onion, peeled
½ a fresh red chilli, deseeded
1 x 450 g jar of roasted red peppers in brine
50 ml white wine
2 x 400 g cans of plum tomatoes balsamic vinegar
150 g smoked mozzarella
12 soft bread rolls

Instructions:
1. Preheat oven to 425ºF.
2. Throw away the crusts from the ciabatta bread. Use your fingers to divide the rest of the bread into bite-sized chunks. Pour cold water over these and set them aside to soak.
3. Mix together the mortadella, mince, eggs, two of the garlic cloves, parsley, and Parmesan cheese. Remove the ciabatta from the water and squeeze out the excess. Add it to this mixture.
4. Get your hands wet and use them to squish the above mixture together until everything is evenly incorporated. Add salt and freshly ground black pepper to taste.

5. Role the mixture into 12 balls and space them evenly on a
baking tray. Spoon a small amount of olive oil over each before putting them in the
refrigerator for approximately 10 minutes.
6. Chop two garlic cloves, chili, and onion. Drain the roasted peppers and chop them as well.
7. Transfer the meatballs from the fridge directly into the oven. Roast them for 15-20 minutes
until slightly browned. Then, transfer them to a large pan over low heat on the stovetop.
8. Pour in the wine and simmer until it reduces. Add onions, chili, and garlic. Cook for 3-5
minutes until the onions brown slightly. Add peppers and the brine from the pepper jar,
chunks of plum tomato, seasonings, and a small amount of balsamic vinegar.
9. Place the pan back in the oven for approximately 25 minutes until the meat is thoroughly
cooked.
10. Slice the mozzarella cheese into 12 pieces and put one on each meatball. Leave them in
the oven just long enough for the cheese to melt.
11. Serve the dish by putting one meatball on each roll with a dollop of tomato sauce and
balsamic vinegar to finish.

Cioppino

Category: Lunch
Difficulty: Easy
Servings: 12
Nutrition facts per serving: 318 Calories
Fat - 12.9g
Carbs - 9.3g
Protein - 34.9g
Cholesterol - 164mg
Sodium - 755 mg

Ingredient List:
3/4 cup butter
2 onions, chopped
2 cloves garlic, minced
1 bunch fresh parsley, chopped
2 (14.5 ounce) cans stewed tomatoes
2 (14.5 ounce) cans chicken broth
2 bay leaves
1 tbsp dried basil
1/2 tsp dried thyme
1/2 tsp dried oregano
1 cup water
1 1/2 cups white wine
1 1/2 pounds large shrimp - peeled and deveined
1 1/2 pounds bay scallops
18 small clams
18 mussels, cleaned and debearded
1 1/2 cups crabmeat
1 1/2 pounds cod fillets, cubed

Instructions:
1. Melt butter in a large pot over medium heat on the stovetop. Stir in chopped onions, minced garlic, and parsley. Stir frequently as the onions become soft.
2. Break up tomatoes from the can and pour them into the pot. Pour in the broth, all spices, wine, and water. Mix and simmer for approximately 30 minutes.
3. Add fish chunks, shrimp, clams, mussels, crabmeat or whatever seafood you chose for the recipe. Increase the heat and allow this mixture to boil. Make sure to cook for 6-8 minutes until all the seafood is cooked through and the clams and mussels open. Discard any shellfish that do not open.

4. Serve in large soup bowls with a hearty bread.

Spinach Salad with Walnuts and Goat Cheese

Category: Salads
Difficulty: Easy
Servings: 2
Nutrition facts per serving: 226 calories
Sugar -1g
Protein - 5g
Dietary Fiber - 3g
Carbohydrates - 8g
Sodium -297mg
Cholesterol - 5mg
Saturated Fat - 3g
Total Fat - 21g

Ingredient List:
Dressing:
1/2 tbsp red wine vinegar
1/2 tbsp shallot or red onion, minced
1 tsp Dijon mustard
1/8 tsp kosher salt
Freshly ground black pepper
1,5 tsp quality walnut oil

Salad:
4 cups baby spinach leaves, trimmed
1/4 cup toasted walnuts, chopped
1/6 cup goat cheese, crumbled

Instructions:
1. Mix together vinegar, mustard, shallots, salt, and fresh ground black pepper. Add oil slowly, whisking the mixture to make it creamy.
2. Toss most of the spinach with the creamy dressing in a large bowl. Add the remainder of the spinach and toss to coat.
3. Sprinkle on crumbled goat cheese and chopped walnuts. Serve right away.

Salsa spaghetti

Category: Dinner
Difficulty: Easy
Servings: 2
Nutrition facts per serving: 414 Calories
Fat -13.2g
Saturated Fat - 2.7g
Protein - 12.9g
Carbs - 64.6g
Sugars - 7.4g
Fibre - 4g

Ingredient List:
160 g dried spaghetti
300 g mixed ripe tomatoes
6 black olives
1/2 bunch of fresh basil
1/2 clove of garlic extra virgin olive oil
1 tbsp red wine vinegar
10 g hard Italian cheese, grated

Instructions:
1. Cook the noodles as directed on the package in a large pan of water for approximately 7-9 minutes. You want your spaghetti to be al dente, which is somewhere between uncooked and mushy.
2. Mix the chopped olives and tomatoes together. Combine this with all but a few of the smallest basil leaves. Also, minced garlic cloves and stirred these in as well.
3. Chop and mash this mixture, or run multiple sharp knives through the bowl until it looks like fresh salsa. Stir in some oil, vinegar, freshly ground black pepper, and salt. Stir until everything is combined perfectly.
4. Drain the spaghetti while saving approximately ½ cup of the water you cooked it in for the sauce.
5. Mix together the pasta, salsa sauce, cooking water, and any additional seasonings you desire. Garnish with the small basil leaves and a sprinkle of grated Parmesan or other hard cheese.

Meal Day 5

Breakfast: Peanut Butter-Banana Muffins – 203 calories
Snack: Healthy Turkey and Tomato Panini – 314 calories
Lunch: Zuppa Toscana – 554 calories
Snack: Red Cabbage Salad – 225 calories
Dinner: Mediterranean Style Fish Gratin – 372 calories

Calories Total Day 5: 1668 calories

Peanut Butter-Banana Muffins

Category: Breakfast
Difficulty: Easy
Servings: 6
Nutrition facts per serving (1 muffin): 203 Calories
Total fat - 9g
Saturated fat - 1.5g
Cholesterol - 15mg
Sodium -280mg
Carbohydrate - 26g
Dietary fiber - 2g
Sugars - 12g
Protein - 6g

Ingredient List:
1/2 cup flour
1/3 cup quick oats, uncooked
1/4 cup sugar
1/2 tbsp baking powder
1/4 tsp salt
1/4 cup creamy peanut butter
1/2 cup milk
1/4 cup ripe banana, mashed
1/2 large egg
1 tbsp oil
1/2 tsp vanilla extract

Instructions:
1. Preheat oven to 375°F.
2. Coat 6 muffin cups with non-stick cooking spray.
3. Mix dry ingredients together.
4. Blend milk and peanut butter until smooth then add banana, egg, vegetable oil, and vanilla extract.
5. Stir blended wet mixture into dry ingredients until moist.
6. Divide mixture evenly into the 6 muffin cups.
7. Bake for 18 to 20 minutes. Insert a toothpick in the center of a muffin. When it pulls out clean, the muffins are done.

Healthy Turkey and Tomato Panini

Category: Appetizers
Difficulty: Easy
Servings: 2
Nutrition facts per serving: 314 Calories
Fat - 8g
Saturated fat - 1g
Fiber- 5g
Carbohydrates - 37g
Protein - 22g
Folate - 10mcg
Cholesterol - 30mg
Sugars - 6g
Sodium - 715mg

Ingredient List:
1,5 tbsp reduced-fat mayonnaise
1 tbsp nonfat plain yogurt
1 tbsp shredded Parmesan cheese
1 tbsp fresh basil, chopped
1/2 tsp lemon juice
Freshly ground pepper, to taste
4 oz thinly sliced reducedsodium deli turkey
4 tomato slices
4 slices whole-wheat bread
1 tsp canola oil

Instructions:
1. Mix mayonnaise, yogurt, cheese, lemon juice, basil leaves, and fresh ground pepper together.
2. Spread this mixture across each piece of bread. Add 1-2 slices of turkey and tomato on top of the sauce mixture. Finish each sandwich with another piece of bread.
3. Turn your stovetop onto medium heat. Add a small amount of healthy oil to a nonstick frying pan.
4. Carefully place each panini in the hot skillet. Fry each side until it is golden brown. This should take approximately 1-3 minutes for each side.
Note: To help the sandwich stay together and the ingredients to blend deliciously, consider using a clean 15- ounce can to weigh down the top of each while you are frying it.

Zuppa Toscana

Category: Lunch
Difficulty: Easy
Servings: 6
Nutrition facts per serving: 554 Calories
Fat - 32.6g
Carbs - 45.8g
Protein - 19.8g
Cholesterol - 99mg

Ingredient List:
1 lb mild Italian sausage
1 1/4 tsp crushed red pepper flakes
4 slices bacon, cut into ½ inch pieces
1 large onion, diced
1 tbsp minced garlic
5 (13.75 ounce) cans chicken broth
6 potatoes, thinly sliced
1 cup heavy cream
1/4 bunch fresh spinach leaves

Instructions:
1. In a Dutch oven or large saucepan, brown the Italian sausage. Add the red pepper flakes to taste during the process. Make sure no pink is left in the meat. This should take 10-15 minutes. Pour off excess fat and put the sausage in another dish for now.
2. Brown the bacon in the same pan. This will take about 10 minutes until all the pieces are crispy. Pour off all but a few tbsp of the fat.
3. Add onions and garlic to the pan and cook until soft. Add the chicken broth and bring the bacon and onion mixture to a boil.
4. Add potatoes and boil for approximately 20 minutes until they are cooked through and soft.
5. Turn the stovetop burner down to medium heat and add the sausage and cream back to the pan. Add spinach leaves directly before you intend to serve the soup.

Red Cabbage Salad

Category: Salads
Difficulty: Easy
Servings: 2
Nutrition facts per serving: 225 calories
Fat - 18.9g
Carbs - 14.6g
Protein - 2g
Cholesterol - 0mg
Sodium - 578mg

Ingredient List:
2,5 Tbsp canola oil
1/4 cup red wine vinegar
1/3 tbsp white sugar
1/3 tsp salt
1/3 tsp seasoned salt
Ground black pepper and onion powder to taste
1/3 head red cabbage, cored and shredded

Instructions:
1. Combine oil, vinegar, sugar, onion powder, salt, and freshly ground black pepper.
2. Stir the dressing over the shredded red cabbage. Allow the salad to rest overnight and drain before serving.

Mediterranean Style Fish Gratin

Category: Dinner
Difficulty: Easy
Servings: 6
Nutrition facts per serving: 372 Calories
Fat - 11g
Saturated Fat - 3g
Carbs - 16g
Sugars - 8g
Fibre - 4g
Protein - 46g

Ingredient List:
3 tbsp olive oil
1 large onion, thinly sliced
1 fennel bulb, thinly sliced
3 large garlic cloves, thinly sliced
1 heaped tsp coriander seeds, lightly crushed
150 ml white wine
2 x 400g cans chopped tomatoes with herbs
2 tbsp tomato purée pinch of saffron
1 bay leaf
1 tbsp fresh lemon juice
1 small bunch flat-leaf parsley, roughly chopped
900g skinless fish fillets, cut into chunks
350g raw king prawn, peeled and deveined

Instructions:
1. Warm up the olive oil in a non-stick frying pan. Add the sliced onion, garlic, and fennel. Sprinkle in the coriander seeds as well. Sauté all of this for approximately 12-15 minutes until everything is tender and begins to turn a golden brown.
2. Add the wine, tomatoes and purée, bay leaf, and saffron to the vegetable mixture. Add salt and pepper if desired and simmer for approximately 12-15 minutes more. The mixture should thicken slightly.
3. Add a large amount of the parsley and lemon juice next. Then, put in the fish chunks and shrimp or prawns. Stir this all together.
4. Put the lid on the pot and simmer everything for approximately five minutes until the fish is cooked. Stir occasionally during the process, but be careful that the chunks of seafood are not broken.

5. Spoon this mixture into six personal-sized casserole dishes. Combine the breadcrumbs, black pepper and
parsley, and cheese.

Meal Day 6

Breakfast: French toast with berry compote – 519 calories
Snack: Bruschetta with tomato and basil – 140 calories
Lunch: Spicy spaghetti vongole – 524 calories
Snack: Grilled Shrimp Skewers on White Bean Salad – 212 calories
Dinner: Wild Mushroom and Barley Risotto – 309 calories

Calories Total Day 6: 1703 calories

French toast with berry compote

Category: Breakfast
Difficulty: Easy
Servings: 2
Nutrition facts per serving: 519 Calories
Fat Total - 19g
Saturated Fat - 10g
Fibre - 5g
Protein - 17g
Cholesterol - 251mg
Sodium - 271.78mg
Sugar - 47g
Carbs - 68g

Ingredient List:
2 eggs
1/6 cup of light cream.
1/6 cup of reduced fat milk.
1/8 cup of caster sugar.
1/2 tsp of ground cinnamon.
15g of butter.
4 slices of thick fruit bread.
100 g of vanilla yoghurt while serving.
Berry compote
1/8 cup of caster sugar.
150g of frozen mixed berries

Instructions:
1. Start by preparing the berry compote. Use a small saucepan and add sugar and 1 tsp cold water.
2. Start heating in low flame till the sugar is dissolved completely.
3. Heat it now till it starts boiling.
4. Continue cooking for 3 minutes till the mixture begins to increase in density.
5. Take it off the flame and add berries, allowing it to cool.
6. Now add cream, milk and eggs in a bowl and mix it thoroughly.
7. Add sugar and cinnamon in a shallow dish.
8. Use a non-stick pan to melt the butter while heating moderately.
9. Dip the bread slices one after the other in the egg mixturetill it soaks.
10. Fry the bread on pan for two minutes till it turns golden brown.

11. After taking the bread off from the pan, toss it in the sugar mixture till it gets coated all over.

12. Keep it covered and warm till you serve it.

13. The toasts taste best when served with yoghurt and compote!

Bruschetta with tomato and basil

Category: Appetizers
Difficulty: Easy
Servings: 2
Nutrition facts per serving: 140 Calories
Fat - 5.1g
Saturated Fat - 0.7g
Protein - 3.2g
Carbs - 20.3g
Sugars - 1.5g
Fibre - 0.8g

Ingredient List:
1 ripe heirloom tomato, chopped
1/3 small bunch fresh basil leaves sea salt freshly ground black pepper
olive oil
white wine or herb vinegar

Instructions:
1. Cut crusty bread into approximately ½ inch thick slices and toast them on the grill or in the pan. Rub each with garlic and sprinkle with top-quality extra-virgin olive oil, and pepper and salt to taste.
2. Clean, trim, and deseed the tomatoes. Chop them into small pieces or pull them apart by hand. Add torn basil leaves, salt, and freshly ground black pepper. Olive oil and vinegar complete the topping for the bread. The seasonings and liquids can be added to taste. I Quality bruschetta is all about the freshest and most delectable toppings. While this recipe sticks with traditional tomatoes and basil, you may also like to try grilled vegetables, artisan cheeses, or a crabmeat salad.

Spicy spaghetti vongole

Category: Lunch
Difficulty: Easy
Servings: 2
Nutrition facts per serving: 524 Calories
Fat - 5.8g
Saturated Fat - 0.7g
Protein - 46.6g
Carbs - 71.3g
Sugars - 4.9g

Ingredient List:
Olive oil
2 cloves of garlic, peeled
150g tin of plum tomatoes
Sea salt
Freshly ground black pepper
150 g spaghetti
1/3 bunch of fresh flat-leaf parsley
1 squid with tentacles, cleaned and sliced
0.5 kg clams, cleaned
35 ml white wine
Extra virgin olive oil
1 fresh red chilies

Instructions:
1. Cook the chili peppers over high heat on a lightly-oiled griddle or grill until their skin is black and crisp. This can also be done over an open flame on a gas burner or grill. It should take about 20 minutes. Set aside to cool in a covered bowl.
2. Peel off the crisp skin of the chilies once they have cooled down enough to handle. Also, remove the stems and seeds.
3. Sauté slices of garlic cloves over low heat in a dollop of oil. Add the chili pieces and tomatoes. Use a wooden spoon or spatula to crush and chop the tomatoes as they cook. Simmer this mixture for 5-7 minutes. Use a potato masher to crush the tomatoes even more and make the sauce smoother. Add salt and freshly ground black pepper to taste.
4. Follow the package directions to cook the spaghetti noodles. Drain them, saving 1 cup of the cooking water, and set the pasta aside.

5. Retain a few parsley leaves for later. Cut up the stalks and the rest of the garlic cloves. Chop the squid tentacles in half and slice the rest of them into smaller pieces.

6. Over medium-high heat, cook the herbs, garlic, wine, a few spoons of the sauce, and the clams together in a large skillet. Toss in the chopped squid and mix well. Cook this all for about 3-5 minutes with a lid on the pot. All the clams should open. If any do not, take them out and discard them.

7. Stir in the rest of the arrabbiata sauce, any additional seasonings, and a drizzle of fresh olive oil. Serve hot right away.

Grilled Shrimp Skewers on White Bean Salad

Category: Salads
Difficulty: Easy
Servings: 2
Nutrition facts per serving: 212 calories
Fat - 8g
Saturated fat - 1g
Fiber - 8g
Carbohydrates - 22g
Protein - 17g,
Folate - 29mcg
Cholesterol - 95mg
Sugars - 2g
Sodium - 575mg

Ingredient List:
1/3 tsp finely grated lemon zest
2 Tbsp cup lemon juice
1 tbsp extra-virgin olive oil
2/3 tbsp packed fresh oregano, minced
2/3 tbsp packed fresh sage, minced
2/3 tbsp minced fresh chives
1/3 tsp freshly ground pepper
Salt to taste
10-ounce cans cannellini beans, rinsed
4 cherry tomatoes, quartered
1/3 cup celery, diced
8 raw shrimp, peeled and deveined (See note.)
Equipment: Two 8 to 10- inch skewers

Instructions:
1. Mix together lemon zest and juice with all the herbs and spices and olive oil. Put aside 2/3 tbsp of this mixture for later.
2. Mix beans, celery chunks, and tomatoes with the remaining dressing until all pieces are well coated.
3. Use a grill or a grilling pan over medium-high heat to cook the shrimp. Rub or brush a thin layer of oil onto the grill or pan beforehand. If necessary, use skewers to control

the shrimp and make it easier to flip them for even cooking. The shrimp should turn out pink and opaque when done.

4. Serve shrimp on a bed of the bean salad with a delicious sprinkle of the dressing you set aside at the start.
Note: If you wish to save the shrimp and salad for 24-48 hours, store them separately in the fridge.
Note: For the most environmentally-conscious meal planning, only buy shrimp certified by an organization like the Wild American Shrimp or Marine Stewardship Council. If not possible, the next best bet are wild harvested shrimp from North America. They are more apt to be collected using sustainable guidelines.
Note: Oiling a grill is easy with a clean paper towel or barbecue brush and a dab of any quality cooking oil.

Wild Mushroom and Barley Risotto

Category: Dinner
Difficulty: Easy
Servings: 2
Nutrition facts per serving: 309 Calories
Fat - 9g
Saturated Fat - 3g
Fiber - 10g
Carbohydrates - 47g
Protein - 9g,
Folate - 39mcg
Cholesterol - 9mg
Sugars - 4g
Sodium - 735mg

Ingredient List:
2 cups vegetable, mushroom or reduced-sodium chicken broth
1/2 cups water
2/3 tbsp extra-virgin olive oil
1/3 small onion, minced
1 clove garlic, minced
1 cups mixed mushrooms, coarsely chopped
1/2 cups pearl barley, rinsed
1/6 cup red wine
2 cups baby arugula
25g cup freshly grated
Parmesan cheese
1/3 tbsp butter
2/3 tsp balsamic vinegar
Freshly ground pepper, to taste

Instructions:
1. Combine the water and broth in a large pot and bring it to a simmer.
2. Turned another burner to medium-high heat and put a bit of oil in a large soup pot or
Dutch oven. Sauté onion and garlic for approximately 2-3 minutes until the onion loses
its opacity. Then, at the mushrooms and sauté them for an additional 2-3 minutes.
3. Pour the barley into the large pot, stirring frequently to incorporate flavors. Use the 1/6
cup of red wine to cook the barley. Also, add about 1/6 cup of the broth. Leave it

simmering until most of the wine is soaked into the grain or evaporated. Then, turn the stove top burner down to medium.

4. Add the remaining broth in increments. Between each addition, wait for the broth to be absorbed until the barley is thoroughly cooked through. This whole process should take approximately 30-45 minutes. At the end, the barley should be firm yet tender and have a creamy consistency. The entire 6 cups of broth may or may not be used.
5. Mix the arugula into the barley mixture after removing the pot from the hot burner. Also incorporate butter, vinegar, and cheese. Add salt and pepper to taste and serve right away.

Meal Day 7

Breakfast: Mushroom Frittata – 122 calories
Snack: Salmon Salad Sandwich – 283 calories
Lunch: Creamy Tomato Chicken with Pasta – 730 calories
Snack: Zucchini or Squash Salad – 165 calories
Dinner: Cannelloni with Spinach and Ricotta – 386 calories

Calories Total Day 7: 1686 calories

Mushroom Frittata

Category: Breakfast
Difficulty: Easy
Servings: 2
Nutrition facts per serving (1 wedge): 122 Calories
Fat - 6.4g
Satfat - 3.2g
Monofat - 2.2g
Polyfat - 0.4g
Protein - 13.3g
Carbohydrate - 3g
Fiber - 0.8g
Cholesterol - 116mg
Iron - 0.9mg
Sodium - 401mg
Calcium - 195mg

Ingredient List:
1/2 packet (approximately 4 ounces) of Exotic mushroom blend
1/4 cup of shredded
Parmigiano-Reggiano cheese
2/3 teaspoon of chopped fresh thyme
1,5 large egg whites
1 large eggs

Instructions:
1. The boiler should be preheated. Use an 4-5 inch skillet that is ovenproof and should be used in medium high heat.
2. The pan should then be coated with a layer of cooking spray.
3. Sauté the mushrooms till the color changes to brown and then, keep the mushrooms somewhere else so that it becomes cool.
4. Use tissues to clean the pan. Now add cheese thyme, mushrooms, 1/8 tsp of black pepper, 1/16 tsp of salt, eggs and egg whites in a bowl and keep stirring continuously.
5. Set the temperature to medium and preheat the oven after using cooking spray on the pan.
6. Now add the mixture of mushrooms and cover it, allowing it to cook for 3 minutes.
7. Once the egg is set, the Mushroom Frittata is ready! Cut into 2 before serving!

Salmon Salad Sandwich

Category: Appetizers
Difficulty: Easy
Servings: 2
Nutrition facts per serving (q Sandwich): 280 Calories
Fat - 9g
Saturated Fat - 3g
Fiber - 4g
Carbohydrates - 29g
Protein - 22g
Folate - 90mcg
Cholesterol - 34mg
Sugars - 3g
Sodium - 607mg

Ingredient List:
7-ounce cans boneless, skinless wild Alaskan salmon, drained
1/8 cup red onion, minced
1 tbsp lemon juice
1/2 tbsp extra-virgin olive oil
1/8 tsp freshly ground pepper
2 tbsp reduced-fat cream cheese
4 slices pumpernickel bread, toasted
4 slices tomato
1 large leaves romaine lettuce, cut in half

Instructions:
1. Mix together canned salmon, minced onion, the lemon juice, ground pepper, and olive oil.
2. On each slice of pumpernickel bread, spread a thin layer of cream cheese.
3. Top the cream cheese with the salmon mixture.
4. Add 2 slices of tomato, a lettuce leaf, and the top piece of bread to serve as sandwiches.

Creamy Tomato Chicken with Pasta

Category: Lunch
Difficulty: Easy
Servings: 3
Nutrition facts per serving: 730 Calories
Total Fat - 20.6g
Saturated Fat - 7.7g
Cholesterol - 100.3mg
Sodium - 223.4mg
Carbohydrate - 99.3g
Dietary Fiber - 15g
Sugars - 5.4g
Protein - 40.2g

Ingredient List:
1 tbsp oil
1 onion, diced
5 cloves garlic, minced
1 can diced tomatoes salt, rosemary, and oregano to taste
1 cup milk or coconut milk
1/2 cup heavy cream or coconut cream
1-2 cups rotisserie chicken, shredded
8 oz gluten-free penne pasta
1/4-1/2 cup shredded sharp cheddar
1 tbsp capers

Instructions:
1. Follow standard directions to cook the pasta and drain it well.
2. Saute garlic and onions in a small amount of oil over medium heat. Add all seasonings and the tomatoes. Keep stirring as these cook together for 3-5 minutes.
3. Pour whatever milk and cream you use into the pan. Simmer for approximately 10 minutes on low heat.
4. Toss the pre-cooked chicken and cheese into the sauce. Heat thoroughly. Mix in the pasta and serve hot with a caper garnish.

Zucchini or Squash Salad

Category: Salads
Difficulty: Easy
Servings: 2
Nutrition facts per serving: 165 calories
Fat - 14.5g
Saturated Fat - 2.2g
Protein - 3.7g
Carbs - 3.8g
Sugars - 3.6g

Ingredient List:
2 courgettes, mixed yellow and green
1/2–1 fresh red chilies
1/2 lemon
Extra virgin olive oil
1/4 tsp mustard powder
Sea salt
Sprigs of fresh basil leaves

Instructions:
1. Peel the courgettes, zucchini, or squash. Use a peeler machine or ribbonizer to make long, thin strands of the vegetables. If you do not have one, cut into thin slices.
2. Chop all the chilies into small pieces and add them to the courgettes.
3. Mix lemon juice, extra-virgin olive oil, mustard powder, and salt in a small bowl or bottle.
4. Pour dressing over vegetables and toss or stir to coat.
5. Serve mixture with thin sliced basil leaves.

Cannelloni with Spinach and Ricotta

Category: Dinner
Difficulty: Easy
Servings: 6
Nutrition facts per serving: 386 Calories
Fat - 16.4g
Saturated Fat - 8.9g
Protein - 21.2g
Carbs - 39.3g
Sugars - 8.8g

Ingredient List:
400 g spinach
Extra-virgin olive oil
1/4 tsp ground nutmeg
1 onion, diced
2 cloves of garlic, smashed
2 X 400 g tins of tomatoes
1 bay leaf
1/2 bunch of basil, leaves picked
1/2 lemon's worth of grated zest
250 g ricotta
1 free-range egg, beaten
2 tsp grated parmesan
150 g cannelloni
2 x 125 g mozzarella balls, sliced

Instructions:
1. Preheat oven to 350°F.
2. Turn on your stovetop burner to low and put oil and spinach in a large pot. Add salt, pepper, and nutmeg until the leaves wilt. Stir occasionally during this process. When the spinach is cooked thoroughly, set it aside to cool.
3. Sauté the onion in a bit of oil until it softens. Then, add tomatoes, garlic, basil, bay leaf, and lemon zest. Simmer this mix for 18-20 minutes until it gets a bit thicker. Add salt and pepper to taste.
4. Squeeze the cooked spinach to get rid of more of the water and juices. Chop it into bite-sized chunks with a sharp knife. Return the leaves to the bowl and mix in the egg, parmesan cheese, and ricotta.

5. Use a wide-mouthed piping bag filled with the spinach mixture to fill the cannelloni tubes. Lay these out in a single layer in a large baking dish.

6. Cover the cannelloni with tomato sauce, chopped basil, slices of mozzarella cheese, olive oil, and any other seasonings you desire.
7. Bake for 40 minutes. The top should begin to brown, but not cook too quickly. If this happens, a loose layer of foil will help. Let the dish set and cool for 5 minutes before serving.

CONCLUSION

Now that we have covered the benefits of following the way the Mediterranean's eat and given you options for meals. Let's now recap what we have learned and learn how to implement it straight away.

The Mediterranean style food is delicious and feels less like a diet than many of the health food choices available. If you haven't heard already, the latest research shows that a diet based on Mediterranean style cooking can reduce the risk of heart disease, stroke and heart attack by as much as thirty percent.

After conducting a study that lasted five years, researchers found that a diet consisting of foods such as olive oil, nuts, produce and fish was significantly more effective in reducing the risk of chronic conditions like stroke and heart disease than a low fat diet. Researchers believe that the combination of nutrient-rich compounds and healthy fats found in Mediterranean style food is what accounts for the benefits to cardiovascular health that they found in the study.

That's good news for you. Mediterranean style food will keep you healthy and, as many others have found, it will help you lose weight as well. It's light on the wallet too. Many of the ingredients such as veggies, nuts, beans, fish and olive oil are inexpensive when compared to other dietary foods. If you have been living on protein bars, juice cleansers, and other supplemental food, then you're in for a surprise when you see how much cheaper Mediterranean style food can be. And, it's delicious too!

Following a Mediterranean diet is simple enough. Just add the following components to your daily routine. - Eat mainly plant-based food. This includes fruit, vegetables, legumes, whole grains and nuts. - Drink a glass of red wine with dinner. No more than seven glasses a week. - Replace butter with extra-virgin olive oil or another source of healthy fats.

- Avoid salt. Use herbs and spices to flavour your food. - Eat more fish and poultry. You should have these at least twice a week but more often is fine.
- Limit your red meat consumption. Red meat is still important, but try to eat it no more than a few times per month. This is a diet that you can follow pretty easily. You can find extra-virgin olive oil in just about every super market along with fresh fruit and vegetables.
If you can, try to obtain fresh fish from a fish market. For poultry and red meat, visit your local butcher to get the healthiest cuts.

I hope you enjoyed this introductory guide to the Mediterranean Diet and now get out there and start living the lifestyle.

BONUS

Preview DASH DIET Cookbook For Beginners

One of the most popular and effective diets next to the Mediterranean diet is the DASH DIET.

Here I share with you the beginning of my introductory DASH DIET book. I convey to you everything you would ever need to know about starting the diet, as well as providing you with a TON of delicious and easy to cook recipes. I've provided the first couple of chapters in this preview, check it out!

If you're interested in the book you can read more about it and/or purchase it on amazon DASH DIET Cookbook For Beginners

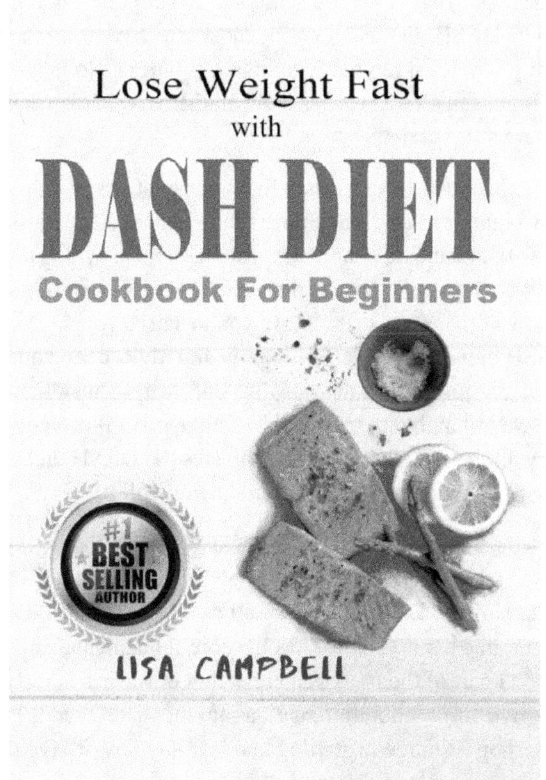

Introduction

The DASH Diet, currently named the healthiest diet in the US, is taking the world by storm, due to its simple, yet effective nature. The DASH diet is special because of its versatility; it can be used to achieve whatever end you are looking for. Looking to be healthier? The DASH diet can reduce your risk of heart disease and lower your blood pressure. Looking to lose some weight? The DASH diet is one of the most effective weight loss diets of the decade, and will easily supercharge your weight loss progress. No matter what your health goals are, the DASH diet can almost certainly fulfill them, which is what makes this diet one of the best diets currently out there.

Since you are reading this book I can assume that you're interested in one of these goals, whether it's to lose weight or to live a healthier life in general. The purpose, and reason why I wrote this book is to educate people like yourself and provide you with the best tools necessary to begin and conquer the DASH diet. The DASH diet is truly a diet that can change your life. Unlike other diets that require you to starve yourself or workout excessively, the DASH diet makes an effort to only slightly change your current lifestyle so that the diet is sustainable for the rest of your life, since eating healthier for a long period of time is the only true way to maintain true health. Unlike other diets, you won't feel restricted and hungry all the time, which is what makes the DASH diet work. When you're finished with the DASH diet you will feel better and you will be better.

The book contains two parts. The first is an all-inclusive guide that will provide with instructions and tips to learn the DASH diet. You will find all you need to know about beginning and maintaining the DASH diet, as well as detailed guides on what to eat and what not to eat. I will discuss the history, as well as the core fundamentals in the DASH philosophy. The second part of the book is a collection of recipes that I've personally tried which I believe will give you a smooth transition into the diet. Overall I hope that this book can be your one stop shop resource to starting and learning how to live the DASH diet lifestyle

CHAPTER ONE:

Everything you need to know about DASH

The DASH Diet – What it's All About?

The History Behind the DASH Diet

The DASH Diet is a revolutionary approach to eating. It's not so much of a diet, but a change of lifestyle geared towards making you a healthier and better individual.

During the past few years, The DASH Diet has been one of the most recommended diets for staying healthy. When DASH was originally created, its purpose was to treat high blood pressure. Hypertension was becoming a large issue in the medical industry, which created a demand for a diet that would work well to help treat these problems. DASH was an immediate success for treating blood pressure, but even though the diet has had great progress for treating medical problems, health organizations soon realized the hidden potential this diet also had for weight loss.

DASH has a long history, so I'll be brief. The diet originated during a series of dietary studies where researchers were trying to discover the best high blood pressure diet by testing out different combinations of foods. The DASH study began in 1993, and went on for 5 years, finally ending in 1997. The studies consisted of three diets, two experimental and one control group. The first experimental group consisted of a high fruit and vegetable diet, and the second group was the DASH diet. The DASH diet group was different from the fruit and veggie group because it also focused on low fat content and high protein and fiber levels. Instead of just eating fruit and vegetables, the DASH diet experiment had participants eating fish, chicken, whole grains, and meats. The Results looked like this:

Diet Group	Effect
Control Group	No Effect
Fruit and Vegetable Diet	Small Positive Effect
DASH Diet	Significant Blood Pressure Drop

Out of the three diets that were running through clinical trials, the DASH diet came out to be the most effective, and showed the most potential to lower blood pressure (11 systolic and 6 diastolic was the average). Researchers immediately studied why this diet was so effective compared to the others they tested. Once they realized the possibility of what they had found they were able to turn their observations into the DASH diet.

At the time the purpose of the research study was only to look at how diet effected blood and therefore didn't focus on weight loss very much. Since the diet was soley going after hypertension the original diet was high in starchy foods and refined grains. Since then, although the basics of the diet have remained the same, it has undergone somewhat of a shakeup. Along the way, research that is more recent has optimized the diet even further, showing even better results than the original research.

The new research has shown that by getting rid of the empty carbohydrates and adding more good lean fats as well as protein, blood pressure could still be improved while at the same time helping the dieter achieve massive weight loss. This is what made the diet such a successful and popular diet.

The letters in DASH stand for **D**ietary **A**pproaches to **S**top **H**ypertension since the original purpose of the diet was to help those who suffer from hypertension. Hypertension is one of the most prominent diseases of our time, and it affects nearly 1 billion people across the world and around 50 million of those in the US alone. High blood pressure can be a serious medical condition due to the correlation between high blood pressure and cardiovascular disease. People with high blood pressure in general will be three times more likely to suffer from a heart attack, as well as a multitude of other undesirable conditions. The higher your blood pressure is, the more chance you have of suffering from a heart attack, stroke, heart failure or kidney disease and, for those within the age range of 40-70, an increase of 20 mm HG in systolic or 10 mm HG in diastolic blood pressure equates to double the risk of cardiovascular disease.

Before the DASH diet, and often times still today, most physicians will tell their patients with high blood pressure to go onto a low sodium diet. Low sodium diets work to reduce blood pressure since salt is a direct contributor to high blood pressure, but overall, a low sodium diet is generally not enough to completely stop hypertension since the body will often adjust to the low sodium diet and again return to having high blood pressure. The DASH diet on the other hand is much more than just a low-sodium diet. It is based on proven research with a plan that involves eating fresh fruit vegetables and low or non-fat dairy. It ditches the refined grains in favor of whole grains and is rich in magnesium, potassium, fiber and calcium. The plan is wholly recommended by: wholly

- The American Heart Association
- The National Heart, Lung and Blood Institute
- The Dietary Guidelines for Americans
- US Guidelines for treating hypertension

Because obesity is on the rise, more and more people are looking for a weight loss diet that really works these days. Thanks to new research done on old data, the DASH diet has been revamped so it not only lowers blood pressure, amongst other things, but it also helps you to drop the pounds, and fast.

DASH Diet in a Nutshell

DASH is pretty easy to follow. It simply focuses on having you eat healthier foods while cutting out foods with high fat content or high carb content, especially refined grains. The major focus for this diet is to eat foods that are rich in vitamins and minerals, foods that have good fats (such as the fats in olive oil), and foods with high fiber content. That's DASH in its simplest form, not so hard to remember.

DASH Diet Essentials

- ✓ Foods with High Vitamins
- ✓ Unsaturated Fat content
- ✓ High Fiber Foods

The biggest DASH diet no no's are foods that are excessively sugary and excessively greasy. DASH promotes the consumption of "good" fatty food but is against the consumption of bad fats, such as trans and saturated fats. Additionally you should heavily cut back on alcohol content and caffeinated beverage consumption, as these are loaded with unnecessary sugars and carbs. Finally, though not as bad as the previously mentioned groups, DASH wants you to limit your starchy food intake. I'll go into much more detail later about exactly where these foods are on the spectrum of EAT to DON'T EAT, but for this section just try to understand the general theory of DASH.

Foods to Avoid or Limit

- ✓ Heavy Greasy Foods (Avoid)
- ✓ Heavy non-Fruit Sugary Foods (Avoid)

✓ Alcohol and Caffeine (Limit)
✓ High Starchy Foods (Limit)

DASH is also trying to lower your blood pressure, and by reducing your sodium intake, your blood pressure will drop automatically, which is great news for those with hypertension. When your blood pressure drops, you instantly benefit from a decrease in the risk of cardiovascular disease and strokes. Because the diet is high in vegetables, fruits and low or non-fat dairy, it is automatically low in cholesterol, sugar and saturated fat. The diet wholly encourages nuts, fish, poultry and grains while discouraging sugary sweets, drinks, high carb foods, processed foods and red meat. It promotes health by including foods that are rich in fiber, calcium, potassium, magnesium and protein. In short, you increase the foods that are good for you and get rid of those that aren't.

The DASH Super Foods

Now that you understand a little of the theory of DASH we can go into a more detail on each of the major food groups and why they're important.

DASH Minerals

One of the key reasons that DASH is able to lower blood pressure is that it contains a high level of minerals, specifically potassium content. DASH also includes minerals such as magnesium and calcium, which are helpful in lowering blood pressure. DASH focuses on obtaining these minerals right from the source, rather than just advocating supplements. Research has found that taking just supplements for mineral intake doesn't have nearly the effect that eating raw fruits and vegetables does, therefore DASH promotes the consumption of minerals through fresh fruits and vegetables. Some studies have even shown that the consumption of supplements on a daily can actually be bad for you.

Fruits and Vegetables

Fruits and vegetables are the core of the DASH diet. Fruits and vegetables are loaded with rich minerals, antioxidants, and a boatload of other healthy nutrients. The DASH diet focuses on consumption of minerals and foods with high fiber, which fruits and vegetables both easily achieve. Fruits are also a great source for water intake, and also can help keep you from having cravings.

When it comes to vegetables, for DASH you want to focus your vegetable consumption on non-starchy vegetables. Starchy vegetables can be good but they contain a lot of sugar when they are processed in the body, which violates our DASH diet rules.

It is recommended that we get around 14grams of fiber for every 1000 calories in our diet. Most people aren't able to achieve this since they don't eat enough whole grain foods or fruits and vegetables. Luckily, with DASH it is easy to get a lot of fiber since most of the foods on the diet are fruits, vegetables, or whole grains. The key to eating fiber on the DASH diet is to make sure you are getting both types of fiber (soluble and insoluble) and not loading up on just one type. Insoluble fiber foods are generally found in whole grain products, while soluble fibers are found in fresh fruits and vegetables. Another major tip for eating a lot of fiber is to make sure you drink a lot of water so that you wont become constipated from too much fiber. Insoluble fiber is helpful for your trips to the bathroom, and can help keep you regular, while soluble fiber can help keep your body healthy by lowering cholesterol and stabilizing your blood sugar. Soluble fiber also assists in keeping you regular and can help intestinal motility. Make sure you check the labels on the foods you purchase, and become well versed with which foods contain which types of fiber, and how much.

Fats and Protein

The DASH diet focuses on minimizing bad fats while promoting good fats. Saturated and trans fats are bad, and should be replaced with a diet consisting of mostly unsaturated fats. One way to try and remember the difference is that saturated and trans fats are mostly solid at cold/room temperatures whereas unsaturated fats are liquid. Butter is a saturated fat and it's solid. Compared to olive oil, which is unsaturated, and liquid at room temperature. Unsaturated fats generally come from lean meats, especially fish, as well as nuts and seeds. Unsaturated fats can actually be beneficial to our health by lowering bad cholesterol and increasing good cholesterol. Make sure you plan on eating several servings of these types of fats. If you don't like eating fish, or can't think of any good foods with good fat content then you may want to consider asking your physician or nutritionist if omega 3 tablets would be a good idea to supplement with your diet.

Make sure you incorporate nuts and beans into your diet, as they are also a great source of these "good fats." Nuts and beans contain heart healthy fats and protein. In a diet where you aren't able to eat fatty meats, it's a good idea to make sure you get a decent amount of protein, and especially if you don't like fish then nuts are a great source. Nuts and beans are also great at keeping you from being hungry, just eating 20 or so can fill you up and keep you occupied until your next meal.

Dairy

Low-Fat and Nonfat dairy are a cornerstone of the DASH diet. One of the reasons why dairy is included is because it has a very significant effect when it comes to reducing blood pressure. Drinking milk alone, not even following the DASH diet can lower your blood pressure by 4-6 points. Dairy is also an extremely important source for calcium and vitamin

D, and the DASH diet is a heavy proponent of vitamins and minerals. If you are lactose intolerant it should be easy to find products that are good substitutes. Make sure you find products that also contain the same nutrition as normal milk, or else substituting would be pointless.

Whole Grains

Whole grains are less important than the other components of DASH, but what makes whole grains important is that whole grains are such a good substitution for refined grains. Whole grains also contain a decent amount of fiber, especially insoluble fiber as well as your primary source for magnesium. Whole grains also have some other vitamins too like vitamin B, but to a lesser degree than fruits and
Vegetables
.

How Does the DASH Diet Work?

The DASH diet is split into 2 phases – the initial weight loss and health phase followed by the maintenance phase. Phase 1 is very similar to many other low carbohydrate diets in that you follow it strictly for 2 weeks. The goal of phase 1 is to help your body transition from normal eating to DASH eating. Phase 1 will help teach your body how to not rely on carbohydrates, since eating high amounts of carbs can cause fluctuating sugar levels, which can often time lead to cravings. Phase 1 helps you to reset your metabolism by dropping wholegrain and fruit from your meals. It is a phase that should see almost instant weight loss results in virtually everyone who does it.

Phase 2 is the maintenance phase and this is where you start to add back in starchy vegetables, fruits and whole grains but slowly so that you can keep an eye on how these reintroduced foods effect your weight, blood pressure and cholesterol levels. In this phase you learn how to eat for the long term, and how to keep your body healthy. I will go into more detailed information about these phases in the next section.

If you want to break down exactly what you should be eating in the DASH diet, you can see that it's highly based in obtaining multiple nutrients and limiting harmful foods. For a person eating 2100 calories per day, the total amount of fat in those calories must not exceed 27% (look at the labels to see how many calories come from fats) and only 6% of that must come from saturated fat. No more than 150 mg of cholesterol must be eaten but 55% of those calories should be in the form of carbohydrates and 18% from protein. Other nutrient goals on a 2100 calorie a day plan include:

- 1250 mg calcium
- 30 g fiber
- 500 mg magnesium
- 4700 mg potassium

- Less than 2300 mg sodium – 1500 is best

Now, this may all seem very complicated but, in truth, it isn't. The following foods are based on a 2000 calorie a day diet and will need to be tweaked depending on your age, activity level and gender. Also keep in mind this is just a guideline:

- **Whole Grains – 6-8 servings per day** - one serving is equal to one slice of bread, ½ cup cooked cereal, rice or pasta, etc. Make sure the food has the word Whole in it, not all brown bread or rice is good for you! Check out the fiber content; look for whole-wheat flour or whole grain flour in the ingredients. Look for grain products that have at least 2 g of fiber in each serving.

- **Fruit – 4-5 servings per day** – one serving equates to a small piece of fruit, 10 grapes, ½ banana, ½ a grapefruit etc. Rather than just eating the fruit as is, add it to your salad or top off your breakfast. Make it your choice for a daily snack as well, rather than a muffin or cookie.

- **Vegetables – 4-5 servings per day** – one serving equals ½ cup of cooked or one cup of raw vegetables. If you don't think you can eat that much in one day, try a few new ways of eating vegetables. Add peppers and tomatoes or spinach leaves to your sandwiches; grill your veggies rather than boiling them. Grilling or roasting really bring out the flavor in vegetables and you retain the nutrients where boiling tends to make foods bland and less nutrient dense.

- **Low or Non-fat Dairy – 2-3 servings per day** – Use skim milk or no higher than 1%. Go for low-fat yoghurts and cheeses. Drink two servings of milk (1 cup each) per day; yoghurt servings are 8 oz. and cheese is 1 oz.

- **Lean Fish, Meat and Poultry – 2 or less servings per day** – Try to eat no more than 6-8 oz. of lean protein per day. Eat fresh chicken leg or breast, turkey breast, pork loin, pork tenderloin, lean cuts of sirloin, ground beef, fresh fish and tinned tuna that is low in sodium.

- **Nuts and Seeds – 4-5 servings per week** - Although these are high in good fat they are also very high in calories. Add a few to your salads or a stir-fry – one serving of nuts is around 1/3 of a cup or 2 tbsp. nut butters. Unsalted seed servings are 2 tbsp.

Healthy Fats – 2-3 servings per day – Use oils that contain monounsaturated fats, like olive oil, peanut oil and canola. Corn and soybean oil contain higher levels of polyunsaturated fats and should also be on your shopping list. Try eating avocado, seeds, olives, natural nut butters, etc., 1 serving of oil or vinaigrette salad dressing is 1 tsp.

Sweets and Fats – 2 or less servings per day – These are foods that you do not need to eat so use this as treats only. Do read the labels to ensure you are eating only one serving, i.e. a 2" brownie square, 1 small donut, 2 small cookies, 8 oz. of sugary soda.

So you can see, there is plenty for you to east, you will never go hungry and it really isn't all that difficult to follow.

Lose Weight with DASH

The DASH diet will automatically jump start your weight loss goals almost regardless of your weight and gender, but to do this more efficiently it's important to understand how many calories you should be eating a day. DASH forces you to eat foods that are rich in minerals and low in fats. Additionally, all of the foods you will be eating on DASH are designed to have a low calorie count while still making you feel full enough that you don't crave extra calories.

In order to determine the general number of calories that you should be eating a day just follow this simple chart. If you are significantly heavier or thinner than the average weight of your age group you might want to consult the Internet or your nutritionist since this chart is just a general guideline. The amount of calories listed on the chart are the calories it takes your body to maintain equilibrium. If you are looking to lose 1 pound a week you should subtract roughly 500 calories from your equilibrium calorie count.

Gender	Age	Sedentary	Moderately Active	Active
Female	18-30	1800-2000	2000-2200	2400
	31-50	1800	2000	2200
	51+	1600	1800	2000-2200
Males	19-30	2400-2600	2600-2800	3000
	31-50	2200-2400	2400-2600	2800-3000
	51+	2000-2200	2200-2400	2400-2800

Sedentary: Defined as normal lifestyle

Moderately Active: Defined as walking 2-3 miles a day or working out every other day

Active Life: someone who walks more than 3 miles a day or who works out dail

CHAPTER TWO:

Everything you need to know about THE DASH DIET PHASES

DASH Diet Phases

I mentioned in the last section that the DASH diet consists of two major phases. This part of the diet is probably the most confusing part since you have to understand how each phase works and follow different foods on each phase. Luckily, the first phase is only 14 days, and the diet never has you shift back to phase one, so once you're finished phase one you only need to adjust to phase two. In this section I'll go over what exactly the purpose of each phase is and what you should eat, as well as what you should avoid.

DASH Diet Phase One

When starting the DASH diet you must spend some time to reset your body so that it can be ready for the diet. Phase one is focused on resetting your metabolism, and helping you become better suited for phase 2. Phase 1 is the more restrictive of the phases, and will help you start your momentum into phase 2. Phase 1 is known to be extremely effective in slimming your waste line since you will be focusing on eating lots of vegetables. People tend to drop the pounds like crazy just by following the first phase of the diet. The key to resetting your metabolism, and purpose of phase 1, is to cut out starchy and sugary foods. Once this occurs your metabolism will operate much better, which will allow you to enter phase 2.

Phase 1 Food Basics

Vegetables

The number one foods for phase 1 (and phase 2) are non-starchy vegetables. Non-Starchy vegetables can be thought of as vegetables that are typically flowering parts of a plant, such as lettuce, broccoli, cucumber, spinach, mushrooms, etc. Starchy vegetables are vegetables such as corn, peas, parsnips, potatoes pumpkins, squash, and zucchini. By avoiding starchy foods you're essentially helping your body to regulate your blood sugar which will diminish your cravings. Starchy vegetables break down into a lot of sugar, which is bad for phase 1 since we are trying to cut down on carbohydrate and sugar dependence. Here is a chart summarizing that

Non-Starchy Vegetables (EAT A LOT)	Starchy Vegetables (AVOID)
Lettuce	Potato
Broccoli	Pumpkin
Cucumber	Corn
Spinach	Green Peas
Mushrooms	Parsnip
Onions	
Peppers	
Tomatoes	
Artichoke	
Asparagus	
Celery	
Daikon	
Eggplant	
Kale	
Leeks	
Salad Greens	
Turnips	
Water Chestnuts	
Radish	
Green Onion	
Snow Peas	

When it comes to non-starchy vegetables you can eat an unlimited amount of these on phase 1. It's actually recommended that you eat at least 5 servings of these vegetables a day, so make sure you're trying your best to find space to eat these during the day. These are your number 1 food for phase 1 so get familiar with them.

Protein and Meat

The next most important food for phase 1 is lean meat. When I say lean meats, I say this because the objective is to get a decent amount of protein intake while limiting fat consumption. For lean meats you should focus on eating things like fish, and poultry. You can also consider things like eggs even though its not meat, but they are a good source of protein.

Lean Meat

Fish
Boneless Skinless Chicken Breast
Eggs
Top Sirloin/Lean Cut Beef
Turkey Cutlets

When it comes to lean meats and protein you should try to eat around 6-8 ounces a day. If you're smaller and eat less, aim for the smaller range of that number, and likewise if you're bigger aim for the larger range.

Everything else

After focusing on the main two food groups of phase one, non-starchy vegetables and lean meat, you can also have some tastes from other food groups, but make sure you limit yourself. In general it's recommended that you have about 2-3 servings of dairy (avoid milk for now), 1-2 servings of legumes, and 2-3 servings of fats.

Foods you can eat but in moderation

Dairy (2-3 Servings)
Nuts and seeds (1-2 servings)
"Good Fats" (2-3 servings)

Unfortunately phase 1 can be a little daunting because of all the foods you have to avoid and limit, but remember its only for 14 days. Here is a chart of foods you should 100% avoid.

Starchy foods (including grains)
Fried Foods
Sugary Foods
Fruit
Alcohol
Milk
Caffeinated beverages
Greasy Foods
Refined Grains and Whole grains

Phase 1 Eating Ideas

Here are some basic ideas for foods during the phase 1 portion of your diet. The first 14 days is pretty tough because you are pretty limited in options, but keep in mind that once you are done it will get easier, also you will lose a ton of weight just from following a strict phase 1 diet for 14 days. It's also recommended that you eat 5 meals a day but keep them small. This will prevent cravings throughout the day because spanning your eating into smaller portions will prevent your body from having huge swings in blood sugar level.

Breakfast Ideas

Hard Boiled Egg
Yogurt
Egg substitute omelets (limit egg consumption to only a few days a week)
Scrambled eggs
1-2 Slices of Canadian Bacon
Tomato juice (Low Sodium)
Cottage cheese

Lunch Ideas

Tuna Salad
Cherry Tomatoes
Small salad with Italian dressing
Sugar free Jell-O
Deli meat rolls (roll up a slice of meat with cheese)
Raw vegetables
Hamburger no bun

Dinner Ideas

Side Salad with balsamic dressing
Broccoli

Roasted turkey
Sautéed vegetables
Grilled Chicken
Raw vegetables

In Between Meal Snacks Ideas

Cheese Wedges
Grape tomatoes
Pepper strips
20 peanuts
Baby carrots
Yogurt
23 Almonds
18 Cashews

Phase 1 Tips

Phase 1 can definitely be tricky, so stay strong and don't lose motivation. The first major tip is to make sure you don't skip any meals. As I mentioned, make sure you are eating around 5 meals a day, breakfast, pre lunch, lunch, pre dinner, and dinner. This will help you reduce cravings that will otherwise push you into eating something spontaneously. Keep your meals light so that each meal is only around 300-400 calories, its better to keep all meals even rather than have breakfast be small and dinner be big. A lot of people believe that skipping meals will make you lose weight faster but in fact it can do the opposite. By skipping meals one of two things can happen 1) your blood sugar level will no longer be steady and you will have cravings and end up eating more 2) your body will slow down its basal metabolism rate, which means fewer calories will keep your body satisfied. In other words, if you ever stop starving yourself you will start to gain weight much faster than before. That's why it's extremely important you do not skip meals.

Some other good tips are to make sure your sleep schedule is steady, go to bed early and make sure you aren't changing your waking and sleep times everyday. In addition to sleeping try and exercise just a little bit but not too much. Go for a 30-minute walk, or use the stairs instead of the elevator at work. You want to make sure your activity level is solid, but you don't want to overdo it during phase 1.

If you decide to dine out during these 14 days there are still several options for you. For breakfast you can order eggs or omelets, as well as some bacon. Remember you cannot have starchy foods so no potatoes or bread. For lunch and dinner a very easy option is to order a salad with oil based dressing. You can add meats and other vegetables to your salads to make them more delicious. You can also order burgers but ask for it without the bun and get it with a side salad instead of fries.

Plan everything during your first week. This will help you to not get demoralized midway through when you don't know what to eat. Bring lunches and extra snacks to work or on long trips and keep this book on hand so you have an easy way to check and see if foods are ok to eat.

Focus on your results during these 14 days. It's very easy to get discouraged when you're starting something new, especially something as life changing as this. Remember that it's only for 14 days and stay positive. Think about the fact that you'll soon lose a good chunk of weight, and that you'll be a step closer to your dieting goals. Never lose hope!

DASH Diet Phase Two

The second phase of the DASH diet puts you into the core food groups of the diet. This phase will add onto what you've learned in phase 1, but will feature more foods that you weren't allowed to eat during the first phase. This phase of the diet should be significantly easier to start than the previous since you are building onto a previously established foundation. There is no time limit to phase 2, so you will be eating from phase 2 foods for the rest of the duration of your diet, which hopefully will be years.

Phase 2 Foods

Good Phase 2 Foods

Just like in phase 1 you'll be able to consume an unlimited quantity of non-starchy vegetables. Turn to these foods whenever you need an idea for a snack, since the more you eat of these the better. Additionally sugar free Jell-O is a great alternative to heavy desserts, and can be eaten almost unlimitedly. Also like in phase 1 you should eat a decent amount of lean meats, as well as foods that are rich in protein and low in fats. Now for phase 2 you will be able to add in fruit, as well as healthy whole grains. These two foods can be eaten moderately, about 2-4 servings a day

The Phase 2 Foods

Non-Starchy Vegetables (Unlimited)
Sugar Free Jell-O (Unlimited)
High Protein Low fat Foods (3-4 servings)
Low Fat/Non Fat Dairy (3-4 Servings)
Fruit (2-4 Servings, limit to 6 servings max)
Nuts (1-2 Servings)
Whole Grains (1-2 Servings)

In phase 2 you are allowed to eat a very limited quantity of refined grains, the recommended amount is a maximum of 3-4 servings each week, but eating 0 is always the best. Save these servings for something you really enjoy to treat yourself, but make sure you don't overdo it because then it will negate the efforts achieved from phase 1. Additionally you want to limit things like heavy sauces (ketchup and BBQ) any foods with trans-fats or high saturated fat content, alcohol, and caffeine.

Starchy Foods
Heavy Sauces, especially high sodium
Foods with Bad Fats (Trans, saturated)
Alcohol
Caffeine
Heavy refined Carbs

Phase 2 Foods to AVOID

Starchy Foods
Heavy Sauces, especially high sodium
Foods with Bad Fats (Trans, saturated)
Alcohol
Caffeine
Heavy refined Carbs

Phase 2 Eating Ideas

Here is a brief list of ideas for meals during phase 2. Now you can have fruits, milk, as well as whole-wheat grains, so the choices are better than for phase 1. For more advanced meal ideas check out the menus in the back of the book.

Breakfast

Eggs
Egg substitute
Canadian Bacon
Juice or Tomato Juice
Yogurt
Milk
Whole Grain Cereal
Fresh fruit
Whole grain oatmeal
Lean meat (small amount of bacon)
Boiled Eggs
Whole grain waffle
  Whole wheat toast
Cheerios

Lunch

Deli Meat rollups
Baby carrots
Fresh Fruit
Salad
Tuna Salad

Chicken Salad
Jell-O
Peanut butter and Jelly Sandwich on whole wheat
Deli sliced sandwich on whole wheat
Cheeseburger with whole wheat bun or no bun
Vegetarian hotdogs
Raw vegetables
Tomato soup (low sodium)

Dinners

Meatloaf
Mashed potatoes
Fish
Whole wheat pasta with meat sauce
Salad with chicken or other lean meat
Chicken Piccata
Green beans and other vegetables
Fruits
Vegetable Lasagna
Greek Salad

Between Meal Snacks

String Cheese
Cherry Tomatoes
Peanuts
Walnuts
Low fat Yogurt
Cashews
Raw Vegetables
Hummus
Baby Carrots
Almonds
Eggs

Phase 2 Summary

Foods to Eat and How much	
Non-Starchy Vegetables	Unlimited
Lean Meat	5-9 ounces
Whole Grains	2-3 servings
Dairy	1-3 servings
Fruits	2-4 servings
Refined Grains	RARE 2-3 times a week
Fats	2-3 servings

If you're interested in the book you can read more about it and/or purchase it on amazon DASH DIET Cookbook For Beginners

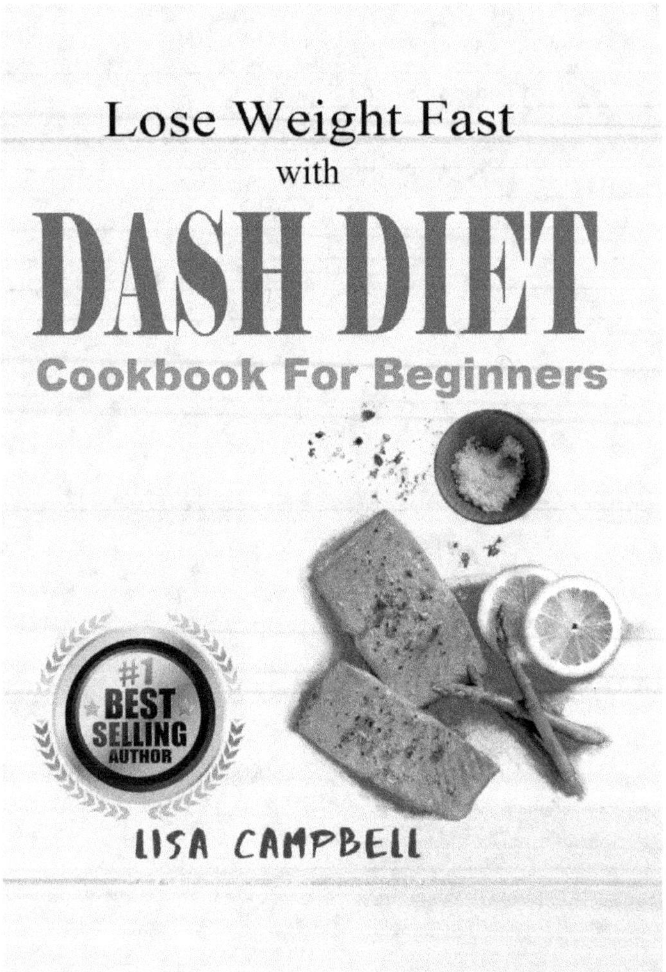